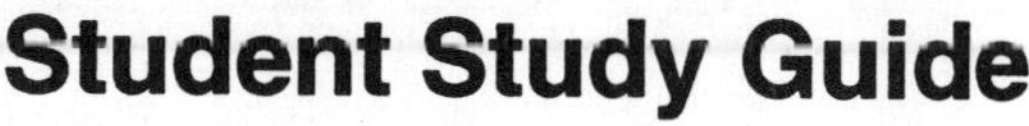

Student Study Guide

to accompany

CONTEMPORARY NUTRITION

Issues and Insights

second edition

GORDON WARDLAW, Ph.D., R.D., L.D.
PAUL INSEL, Ph.D.
MARCIA SEYLER, M.Phil.

Prepared by

Gordon Wardlaw, Ph.D., R.D., L.D.
Division of Medical Dietetics
The Ohio State University

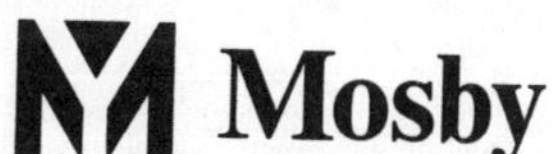

Mosby

St. Louis Baltimore Boston Chicago London Madrid Philadelphia Sydney Toronto

PREFACE

Mastering Nutrition

I found four important methods for learning course material and making good examination scores when I was a student. I advise you to do all four. This <u>Study Guide</u> to accompany <u>Contemporary Nutrition: Issues and Insights</u> is designed to help you with the last three.

1. Attend every class period. This is vital because no book or study guide can substitute for a clear explanation of a term or concept by a professor. In addition, although examinations are based on factual material, they also are greatly influenced by the professor's frame of mind. The student needs to both understand important concepts, and also categorize those concepts in terms of the relative importance the professor puts on them.

2. Read the textbook. You should spend at least one hour outside of class for every hour in class reading your textbook. Underline important points. Write in the margins. Use the book to help you understand the concepts developed in class. Follow along in the <u>Study Guide</u> to practice using those concepts. Ideally, read the relevant sections in the textbook and <u>Study Guide</u> before going to class. You will find that a very helpful exercise.

3. Use flash cards. A flash card has a word or concept on one side and a corresponding definition or explanation of the concept on the other side. Using flash cards is a powerful method for learning material because you cannot fool yourself into thinking you know the material. Either you know what's on the other side of that flash card - or you do not. Simply reading your notes or looking at the underlined sections of your book is not enough. In my 15 years of teaching I have seen students increase their grades significantly once they started using flash cards. I used this system throughout my undergraduate and graduate course work. I even convinced many of my friends in graduate school to use this technique.

I have included a group of flash cards for every chapter in this <u>Study Guide</u>. Providing information in this form is a key part of the approach this guide takes. These are just a start. Make more flash cards for other concepts you think are important. Review your flash cards every day or two. Before an examination review all of them until you know each one. Before the final examination sit in a chair next to a trash can. Run through your flash cards and discard every one you know, and then keep running through the remainder until all are in the trash. In that way you have efficiently reviewed material from the entire course, and are ready to excel in the final examination.

4. Take practice examination. I always found it helpful to take as many previous examinations from a class as I could. These helped me get into the rhythm of taking tests in that subject and challenged me to apply the terms and concepts I had learned. The practice setting allowed time to look up questions I could not answer. I strove eventually to score all answers correctly.

This <u>Study Guide</u> includes about 25 practice examination questions per chapter. Consider making up more of your own. It is important not to simply memorize an answer but to understand why an answer is correct <u>and why the others are wrong.</u> In that way practice questions will challenge you to apply the concepts you have learned.

This <u>Study Guide</u> has four major sections for each chapter. First, objectives for the chapter are listed to help focus your attention while reading the chapter. Then important word parts are given to help you master the vocabulary. Next you should review the flash cards (see Appendix A) to reinforce the most important chapter concepts. The review and synthesis activities then help reinforce the chapter concepts as you study chapter Tables and Figures, provide short answers to questions, perform calculations, and analyze aspects of your diet. Finally, examination questions test you over the terms and concepts in the chapter. Since classroom examinations usually cover four to six chapters, the <u>Study Guide</u> will provide you with about 100-150 sample test questions for each examination.

In all, I think that this <u>Study Guide</u> has a system that will help you learn the text material and do well on examinations. This guide is <u>not</u> a short cut for learning nutrition or a substitute for reading the textbook or attending class. It does, however, provide a logical means by which to study the material, and in turn excel in the class.

CONTENTS

CHAPTER 1
What You Eat and Why

Begin each new Chapter by reading it straight through, while striving to master the following points. Then, start your <u>Study Guide</u> activities.

I.   **Points to consider**

Chapter 1 is designed to allow you to:

1.   Define the terms carbohydrate, protein, lipid (fat), alcohol, vitamin, mineral, kcalorie, and dietary fiber.

2.   Outline the ABCD of nutrition assessment: <u>a</u>nthropometric, <u>b</u>iochemical, <u>c</u>linical, and <u>d</u>ietary.

3.   List the major characteristics of the American diet and the areas that often need improvement.

4.   Describe how various factors affect our food habits: early experiences, ethnic customs, health concerns, advertising, social class, and economics.

5.   Outline the basic units used in the metric system and interpret a percentage value.

II.   **Word parts**

Complete the following exercise using words from Chapter 1 for the examples. This will help you master nutrition vocabulary.

Word Part	Meaning	Examples
hydr	water	__________
bi(o)	life	__________
anthrop	man	__________
metr	measure	__________
kilo	1000 times	__________
centi	100 times	__________
milli	1/1000	__________

III.   **Flash cards**

Cut out and review the flash cards for this chapter in Appendix A.
These will help you focus on the major points of each chapter.

IV.   **Review and synthesis**

These exercises provide an opportunity for you to practice using knowledge gained from lectures, the textbook, and the flash cards. Check your answers to the questions using the page references for your textbook (in parentheses). Some answers also will be listed near the end of the chapter in this <u>Study Guide</u>. This will be pointed out to you when that is the case.

A.   "You have probably heard the terms carbohydrates, protein, lipids (fats and oils), vitamins, minerals. These, plus water, make up the six classes of nutrients found in food." From memory, list some of the essential nutrients in the human diet and their approximate contribution to body weight under the correct category. (6)

	ENERGY NUTRIENTS				
Carbohydrate	Fat	Protein (amino acids)	Vitamins	Minerals	Water

.

Percentage
of body
weight

Refer to Table 1-2 in your text to check your answers, and then use the chapter to add any missing information. Review this exercise again during the next few weeks to refresh your memory.
Check your answers and then add any missing information.

B.   1.   "Energy is held in the chemical bonds of carbohydrates, fats, proteins, and alcohol." Briefly characterize the energy sources in a diet. Then complete the rest of the table. (12)

Energy source	Kcals per gram	Percentage of kcals in U.S. diet
Carbohydrate		
Protein		
Fat		
Alcohol		too variable between individuals

2.   "To figure out how many kcalories are in a particular food portion, we would need to use an instrument called a bomb calorimeter." Describe how a bomb calorimeter works. (12)

3.   A piña colada drink may have 15 grams of alcohol, 6 grams of carbohydrate, 1 gram of fat, and 1 gram of protein. How many kcalories would it contain?

Check your answer on page 16 in this <u>Study Guide</u>.

C.   "Good nutrition and health habits can help maximize health and reduce the chances of developing nutrition-related diseases. Choices you make concerning diet, exercise, and lifestyle all contribute to this goal." List one practice that may prevent the following ill-health outcomes. (12)

Disease condition	Preventive nutrition and health practice
Hypertension	
Liver disease	
Anemia	
Birth defects	
Nutrient toxicities	
Obesity	
Premature heart disease	
Bone loss	
Non-insulin dependent diabetes	

D.   1.   "Anthropometry, biochemical, clinical, and dietary evaluations make up the ABCD of nutrition assessment." Describe what the following components of a nutrition assessment represent. (10)

Anthropometric assessment

Biochemical (laboratory) assessment

Clinical assessment

Diet history

2.	"Food symbolizes much of what we think about ourselves." Provide two examples of this from your life, while discussing the most important determinants of the foods you eat. (You listed these in the Rate Your Plate activity in Chapter 1). (17)

E.	"As people migrate, their cuisines tend to meld together into combinations of other diets and their own." Discuss how various ethnic cuisines have influenced your diet. For example, consider how regularly you eat pizza, tacos, burritos, fried rice, egg rolls, and gyros. (19)

V.   Applying nutrition to your life

"You will use a few mathematical concepts in studying nutrition. Besides performing addition, subtraction, multiplication, and division you need to know how to calculate percentages and convert English units of measure to metric units." The following exercise will allow you to practice math skills for nutrition. (8)

A.   Jim typically has little time in the morning to prepare his favorite breakfast of an omelette, bacon, and biscuits. Instead, he usually relies on a few quick handfuls (1 ounce) of dry cereal to satisfy his hunger. Using the Table of U.S. RDAs (soon to be renamed (RDIs)) and the cereal label provided below, calculate the <u>missing amounts</u> of the specified nutrients he consumes.

Nutrient	U.S. RDA (RDI) (milligrams)	
vitamin C	60	milligrams
thiamin	1.5	milligrams
niacin	20	milligrams
calcium	1000	milligrams
iron	18	milligrams

Cereal Label

Nutrients	milligrams in 1 oz. of cereal	% of U.S. RDA (RDI)
vitamin C	15 milligrams	------
thiamin	------	25%
niacin	5 milligrams	------
calcium	60 milligrams	------
iron	------	25%

B.   Now practice a few metric and English conversions to fine-tune your nutrition math skills:

1 meter	= ______________	inches
1 inch	= ______________	centimeters
1 ounce	= ______________	grams
1 kilogram	= ______________	pounds
1 teaspoon	= ______________	milliliters
1 cup	= ______________	milliliters
1 cup	= ______________	tablespoons
1 quart	= ______________	cups
1 tablespoon	= ______________	teaspoons

1.   A 6'2" man weighs 185 pounds. Change to centimeters and kilograms.

____

2.   If you eat a chicken breast that is 4-1/2 ounces, how many grams did you eat?

____

3.   If you drank 360 milliliters of milk, how many cups did you drink?

____

4.   A tablespoon of pureed infant food equals how many teaspoons?

____

5.   How many quarts of milk did you drink in question #3?

____

Check your answers on page 16 of this <u>Study Guide</u>.

This exercise will pull together the major concepts from the chapter.
Fill in the blanks using the words listed at the end of this summary.

Nutrition is the study of the __________ vital for health and how the body uses these to promote and support __________, maintenance, and __________ of cells. The nutrients in foods fall into six classes: __________, lipids (fat and oils), __________, vitamins, minerals, and __________. The first three, along with alcohol, provide __________ for the body to use. A basic plan for health promotion and disease prevention includes eating a proper diet, __________ regularly, not smoking, limiting alcohol intake, limiting stress, and consulting health care professionals when necessary. Good nutrition should be based on eating the right food, not on taking __________. This strategy supplies nutrient needs, and essentially eliminates the possibility of __________. Results from large nutrition surveys in the United States suggest that some Americans need to concentrate on consuming foods that supply more vitamin A, __________, vitamin B-6, __________, magnesium, iron, __________, and dietary fiber.

Our food choices are greatly affected by our __________, our family, our upbringing, our __________, and the image we want to present to others. __________ influences on the diets of many Americans are notable. A simple, healthful diet is the __________ food for people who live close to the land, such as is true in much of Mexico and __________. They eat a diet based on a grain, fruits, and vegetables, small amounts of dairy products, or meat, fish, eggs, and a type of pea or __________. These diets are healthful because they are low in __________ and high in __________.

Use the following words to complete the summary

bean	exercising	supplements
calcium	fat	traditional
carbohydrates	food	vitamin C
China	growth	water
culture	nutrient imbalances	zinc
dietary fiber	proteins	
energy	reproduction	
ethnic	self-image	

Check your answers using the summary for Chapter 1 in your textbook, and the next page of this <u>Study Guide</u> for the last five answers.

Answers to selected questions

IV. B.3. Piña colada = (15 x 7) + (6 x 4) + (1 x 9) + (1 x 4) = 142 kcalories

V. A.   25%; 0.375; 25%; 6%; 4.5

   B.   39; 2.5; 28; 2.2; 5; 240; 16; 4; 3; 188/84; 126; 1.5; 3; 0.375

VI.   ethnic; traditional; China; bean; fat; dietary fiber

VII.   Practice examination

Use this examination to test your knowledge. Cover the answers on your initial attempt.

Match the chronic disease to the possible cause:

C	1.	heart disease
E	2.	stroke
A	3.	hypertension
D	4.	adult-onset diabetes mellitus
B	5.	cirrhosis of the liver

A. excess sodium intake
B. long-standing alcohol intake
C. poor blood flow in the heart
D. poor insulin function caused by obesity
E. blood clot in the brain

  C 6.   A function of carbohydrates in the diet is to:

    A. absorb and transport vitamins.
    B. promote growth and repair of tissues.
    C. supply energy.
    D. allow for enzyme action.

  C 7.   Good sources of carbohydrate are:

    A. fats, oils, butter, and margarine.
    B. fish, eggs, beef, pork, and poultry.
    C. cereals, fruits, vegetables, and milk.
    D. green leafy vegetables, seafood, and water.

  A 8.   Functions of lipids in the diet are to:

    A. provide fats essential for body function.
    B. transport water-soluble vitamins.
    C. promote growth and repair of tissue.
    D. maintain fluid balance.

  A 9.   Lipids are supplied in large quantities in the diet by:

    A. fats, oils, meats, and nuts.
    B. cereals, fruits, vegetables, and breads.
    C. deep green and orange vegetables, and citrus fruits.
    D. green pepper, broccoli, cantaloupe, and citrus fruits.

| B | 10. | A function of protein is to: |

A. provide essential fatty acids.
B. promote growth and repair of the body.
C. make sex hormones.
D. prevent cell damage.

| D | 11. | Good sources of protein in the diet are: |

A. fats, oils, butter, and margarine.
B. green pepper, cantaloupe, citrus fruits, and broccoli.
C. deep green and orange vegetables, and citrus fruits.
D. meats, fish, legumes, nuts, dairy products, and eggs.

| B | 12. | Essential nutrients: |

A. are made by the body.
B. must be supplied by food.
C. include alcohol.
D. are enzymes.

| B | 13. | A kcalorie is a: |

A. measure of fat weight.
B. unit for expressing energy content in food.
C. scientific instrument.
D. term used to describe the amount of sugar and fat in a food.

| D | 14. | Food likes and dislikes are affected by our senses. |

In describing sensory responses to food, which term does not fit?

A. taste   C. sight
B. smell   D. nutritional value

| A | 15. | The building blocks of proteins are: |

A. amino acids.
B. fatty acids.
C. glucose units.
D. coenzymes.

| C | 16. | Of the following the most concentrated source of kcalories is: |

A. starch.
B. protein.
C. alcohol.
D. sugar.

| C | 17. | Which of the following is the correct number of essential nutrients for humans? |

A. 5 to 10   C. 40 to 50
B. 15 to 20   D. 70 to 80

| C | 18. | The amount of fat in the human body is: |

A. 13% of body weight.
B. 70% of body weight.
C. varies greatly between individuals, but is often higher in women.
D. equals the weight of the muscle tissue.

__D__   **19.**   To promote a nutritious diet, one should keep in mind:

A. variety.
B. moderation.
C. balance.
D. all of the above.

__D__   **20.**   Which of the following would not be included in anthropometric measurements?

A. height and weight.
B. head circumference.
C. skinfold thickness.
D. blood and urine tests.

__B__   **21.**   A slice of bread with 1 gram of fat, 10 grams of carbohydrate, and 2 grams of protein contains:

A. 42 kcalories.
B. 57 kcalories.
C. 82 kcalories.
D. 102 kcalories.

__D__   **22.**   Nutrients that supply kcalories are:

A. fats and vitamins.
B. minerals and water.
C. minerals and vitamins.
D. fats and carbohydrates.

__B__   **23.**   Blacks often need to pay special attention to the amount of salt in their diet because they have a much greater chance of developing:

A. cancer.
B. hypertension.
C. cardiovascular disease.
D. diabetes mellitus.

__B__   **24.**   Diets of rural peoples are characteristically low in:

A. fiber.
B. fat.
C. protein.
D. starches.

__C__   **25.**   The science of food; the nutrients and substances therein; their action, interaction, and balance in relation to health and disease is a definition of:

A. life.
B. energy metabolism.
C. nutrition.
D. food science.

Chapter 2
Tools for Diet Design

I.   **Points to consider**

Chapter 2 is designed to allow you to:

1.   Describe the states of nutritional health varying from overnutrition to a clinical lesion.

2.   Describe what the Recommended Dietary Allowances (RDAs) represent and explain why all essential nutrients do not have an RDA.

3.   Describe the Food Guide Pyramid.

4.   Identify where one can obtain reliable nutrition advice.

5.   List the Dietary Guidelines and the diseases these Guidelines are designed to prevent or minimize.

6.   Describe what a nutrition label consists of and how one can be used to evaluate a food choice.

II.   **Word parts**

Complete the following exercise using words in Chapter 2.

Word Part	Meaning	Examples
is or iso	same	__________
chron	time	__________
chole	bile	__________
osis	disease	__________
scler	hard	__________
vita	life	__________

III.   **Flash cards**

Cut out and review the flash cards for this chapter in Appendix A.

IV.   **Review and synthesis**

A.   "You reach a desirable amount of a particular nutrient when the body tissues have enough of that nutrient for both routine chemical processes and surplus stores." Describe what the following levels of nutritional status represent and provide an example of each concept using iron storage in the body. (34)

General condition	Condition with respect to iron storage in the body
Desired nutritional state	
Undernutrition	
Body deficiency	
Clinical symptoms	
Overnutrition	

B.   1.   "Many men were rejected from military service during World War II because of the effects of poor nutrition on their health." How should the RDAs be properly applied? (36)

    If your dietary intake is less than the RDA for a nutrient, do you necessarily have a deficient diet? Why? (37)

    2.   "The Food and Nutrition Board sets Estimated Safe and Adequate Daily Dietary Intakes (ESADDI) for several nutrients that have no true RDA." List four vitamins and/or minerals for which only estimated safe and adequate intakes have been established. (38)

    a.   c.

    b.   d.

C. "A regular intake of protein is critical to maintain health." The RDA for protein for adults is 0.8 grams per kilogram of one's desirable body weight. (Remember 1 kilogram = 2.2 pounds). Complete the following exercise in relation to protein needed for a 42 year old male who weighs 172 pounds. (37)

Person's RDA for protein:

Possible protein food sources:

Symptoms of protein deficiency:

<u>Define:</u> positive protein balance

protein equilibrium

negative protein balance

D. 1. "One practical application of the RDA are the U.S. Recommended Daily Allowances (U.S. RDA)." Compare the RDA and the U.S. RDA for your age and gender for vitamin A, vitamin E, calcium, and iron. Which of these RDA are quite different than the U.S. RDA? (see the inside cover and Appendix E in your textbook). (39)

a. vitamin A c. calcium

b. vitamin E d. iron

2. In what circumstances is the U.S. RDA used?

3. What are the Reference Daily Intakes (RDIs), and on what are they based?

4. Daily Reference Values (DRVs) serve what purpose?

E.　　1.　　"In the 1940s, nutritionists began to translate the RDA into more practical terms."
Complete the Food Guide Pyramid summary based on adult recommendations. (44)

Food Group	Servings	Major Nutrients	Examples of Food Choices
Milk, yogurt, and cheese			milk, cheese, yogurt, cottage cheese, custard/pudding, and ice cream
Meat, poultry, fish, dry beans, eggs, and nuts			cooked meat, poultry, fish, cooked dry beans, and eggs
Fruits			cooked fruit, fruit juices, fresh fruits, and salads
Vegetables			raw vegetables, cooked vegetables, vegetable juices
Breads, cereals, rice, and pasta			bread, ready-to-eat cereal, cooked cereal, rice, or pasta
Fats, oils, and sweets			margarine, vegetable oil, candy bars

2. "The foundations of nutrition are variety, balance, and moderation." Describe how to use the Food Guide Pyramid. What are two of its strengths and two of its weaknesses? (45)

F. 1. "Most of the major chronic 'killer' diseases in the United States are not associated with deficiencies in protein, vitamins, or minerals." List the Dietary Guidelines for Americans. Next to each Guideline list a specific disease being addressed. (47)

a.

b.

c.

d.

e.

f.

g.

2. "Dietary advice has been issued by various private and governmental organizations."
    Table 2-5 gives some advice for applying dietary guidelines to one's own diet. Practice
    alternating some food habits you want to change by substituting more healthful options.
    (51)

<u>Your typical food choices</u>   <u>More healthful options</u>

a.

b.

c.

d.

e.

f.

g.

h.

i.

j.

3. Describe briefly how the Exchange System differs from the Food Guide Pyramid and the
    Dietary Guidelines in terms of tools for diet planning. (54)

G.	"Food markets are happy to satisfy our craving for health foods with healthy-sounding choices labeled no cholesterol, low fat, organic, and sugar free." However, the terminology used is often misleading. The following exercise tests your ability to identify the vocabulary that is typically confusing. (61)

Match the following words with the definitions below.

_____ sodium free _____ low cholesterol _____ fortified
_____ no cholesterol _____ dietetic _____ no artificial coloring
_____ very low sodium _____ imitation _____ low sodium
_____ enriched _____ cholesterol free _____ sugar free

A.	The product contains no more than 35 milligrams of sodium per serving.

B.	This product does not contain sucrose, honey, fruit juice, molasses, or other simple sugar.

C.	The product contains 20 milligrams or less of cholesterol per serving.

D.	A product that contains no more than 40 kcalories per serving or at least one third fewer kcalories than the regular product.

E.	The vitamins thiamin, riboflavin, niacin, and the mineral iron have been added to the product to replace what is lost in processing.

F.	A product that does not follow the usual recipe for that type of product. Such products may also be lower in nutrients, such as protein, vitamins, and minerals.

G.	Vitamins and/or minerals that were not originally present have been added to the product.

H.	The product contains no cholesterol.

I.	This product contains no more than 5 milligrams of sodium per serving.

J.	The products contain colors from naturally occurring products, such as beet juice, grape skins, or carrot oil.

K.	The product contains less than 2 milligrams of cholesterol per serving.

L.	The product contains no more than 140 milligrams of sodium per serving.

V.   Applying nutrition to your life

"Foods packaged and sold in the United States are labeled." Answer the following questions about "Wheat and Raisins" based on the label. (38)

A.   Traditional nutrition label

<u>"WHEAT AND RAISINS"</u>

NUTRITION INFORMATION
  PER SERVING

	1 oz.
Serving size.....1 ounce (3/4 cup)	
Servings per package	18
Kcalories	110
Protein, g	2
Carbohydrate, g	23
Fat, g	1
Cholesterol, mg	0
Sodium, mg	140
Potassium, mg	100

PERCENTAGE OF U.S. RECOMMENDED
  DAILY ALLOWANCES (U.S.RDA)

Protein	2
Vitamin A	25
Vitamin C	*
Thiamin	25
Riboflavin	25
Niacin	25
Calcium	4
Iron	25
Vitamin D	*
Vitamin B-6	25
Folic Acid	25
Phosphorus	8
Magnesium	4
Zinc	2
Copper	4

*Contains less than 2 percent of
the U.S. RDA of this nutrient.

  INGREDIENTS:

Whole wheat, raisins, sugar, honey,
brown sugar syrup, salt, cereal
malt syrup, calcium carbonate,
trisodium phosphate, a B vitamin
(niacinamide), iron (a mineral
nutrient), annatto extract color,
vitamin A (palmitate) vitamin B-6
(pyridoxine hydrochloride),
vitamin B-2 (riboflavin), vitamin
B-1 (thiamin mononitrate),
A B vitamin (folic acid).

CAPTAIN MILLS, INC.
ST. PAUL, MINNESOTA 55440
Made in U.S.A.

What portion size would yield
55 kcalories?

What percentage of kcalories in a serving is carbohydrate?

How much vitamin A does one serving
yield (U.S. RDA is 5000 IU)?

How much magnesium does one serving
yield (U.S. RDA is 400 milligrams)?

What ingredient is in the greatest
amount, based on weight?

How many forms of sweeteners do you see in
this product?

Where could you write to either
find more information about this
product or file a complaint?

Check your answers on page 30 of this <u>Study Guide</u>.

B.   New nutrition label

"WHEAT AND RAISINS"

NUTRITION FACTS

Serving Size 3/4 cup (24 g)
Servings Per Container 18

AMOUNT PER SERVING
Calories 110   Calories from Fat 9%

	% Daily Value
Total Fat 1 g	2%
Saturated Fat 0.5 g	3%
Cholesterol 0 mg	0%
Sodium 140 mg	6%
Total Carbohydrate 23 g	8%
Sugars 5 g	
Dietary Fiber 3 g	12%
Protein 2 g	

Vitamin A 25% Vitamin C 2% Calcium 4%
Iron 25%

*Percents (%) of a Daily Value are based
on a 2,000 calorie diet. Your Daily Values may
vary higher or lower depending on your calorie
needs:

Nutrient	2,000 Calories	2,500 Calories
Total Fat Less than	65g	80g
Sat Fat Less than	20g	25g
Cholesterol Less than	300 mg	300 mg
Sodium Less than	2,400 mg	2,400 mg
Total Carbohydrate	300g	375g
Fiber	25g	30g

INGREDIENTS:
Whole wheat, raisins, sugar, honey,
brown sugar syrup, salt, cereal
malt syrup, calcium carbonate,
trisodium phosphate, a B vitamin
(niacinamide), iron (a mineral
nutrient), annatto extract color,
vitamin A (palmitate) vitamin B-6
(pyridoxine hydrochloride),
vitamin B-2 (riboflavin), vitamin
B-1 (thiamin mononitrate),
A B vitamin (folic acid).

CAPTAIN MILLS, INC.
ST. PAUL, MINNESOTA 55440
Made in U.S.A.

Briefly explain what Daily Value represents.

Why are only a few vitamins and minerals listed?
Are the others simply not present?

Many of the values are based on Daily Reference Values (DRVs).
What do the DRVs represent?
Are these the same as RDAs?

VI.   Chapter 2 summary

Fill in the blanks using the words listed at the end of this summary.

As nutritional health diminishes, nutrient __________ in the body are depleted. __________ in the body then slow down. Finally, outward __________ symptoms appear.

Recommended Dietary Allowances are set for many nutrients. These levels represent the amount of a __________ that healthy people should consume regularly to meet their needs for that nutrient. The U.S. RDA guidelines differ for men and women, and for various __________ groups.

The __________ is based primarily on the highest RDA levels found in the 1968 publication. The RDA forms the basis for listing nutrients on __________. As part of new government regulations, the U.S. RDAs will soon be replaced by __________. __________ will also be set for other nutrients and combined under a category called __________.

The Food Guide Pyramid provides a way to turn nutrients recommendations from the RDA into a __________. This guide emphasizes __________ milk products, proteins from vegetables as well as from __________; citrus fruits, __________ vegetables, and whole-grain breads and cereals.

The Dietary Guidelines help one to plan a menu pattern to reduce risks of developing __________ diseases. These guidelines emphasize eating a __________ of foods, maintaining a desirable body weight, and limiting intake of __________, cholesterol, __________, and alcohol, while including ample fruits, vegetables, and __________.

Nutrient density reflects the nutrient content of food in relation to its __________ content. Nutrient-dense foods are __________ in nutrients compared to energy content. The __________ system provides a powerful tool for estimating the carbohydrates, fat, protein, and kcalorie content of a food or meal.

A __________ can help fine-tune dietary advice into a custom diet plan to meet your particular health needs and _________.

Foods packaged and sold in any United States supermarket usually are labeled with the _____________, the manufacturer's name and address, the amount of product in the package, and the ___________ listed in order of amount from most to least by __________. Since 1973, if a manufacturer adds a nutrient to a food product or makes a nutritional claim about the product, a _____________ must also be provided. This lists the serving size of the product, the number of servings per package, and many nutrient amounts per serving. Soon almost all _________ will carry such a label.

Use the following words to complete the summary.

age	foods	product name
biochemical reactions	grains	RDIs
chronic	food labels	Registered Dietitian
clinical	food plan	rich
Daily Values (DVs)	ingredients	salt
dark green	lean meat	stores
DRVs	lifestyle	U.S. RDA
energy	low fat	variety
exchange	nutrient	weight
fats	nutritional label	

Check your answers using the summary for Chapter 2 in your textbook and the next page of this <u>Study Guide</u> for the last five answers.

V. serving = 3/8 cup; amount of vitamin A = 0.25 x 5000 = 1250 IU; (23 x 4)/110 = .86 or 86% carbohydrate; amount of magnesium = 0.04 x 400 = 16 milligrams; whole wheat is in greatest amount (first ingredient); 4 sources -- sugar, honey, and both syrups; Captain Mills is the manufacturer

VI. Registered Dietitian, product name, ingredients, weight, nutrition label

---

VII. Practice examination

Cover the answers on your initial attempt.

__A__ 1. The RDA are nutrient levels:

A. used as guidelines for diet planning for groups.
B. that ensure good health for all individuals.
C. that represent minimum daily needs.
D. All of the above.

__B__ 2. If your daily intake of a vitamin does not meet the RDA:

A. you necessarily have a poor diet.
B. you may not be meeting your needs.
C. this is of no consequence because the RDA are designed for groups.
D. you are safe if you meet at least half the RDA.

__B__ 3. A nutrition label listing selected vitamin and mineral contents must appear if:

A. a vitamin or mineral has been lost in processing.
B. the manufacturer advertises the nutritional benefits for the food.
C. the food uses "enriched" flour.
D. the food does not have a Standard of Identity.

__A__ 4. "Enriched" grains do <u>NOT</u> have which one of the following substances added back?

A. fiber   C. iron
B. niacin   D. thiamin

__D__ 5. One of the following is <u>NOT</u> a U.S. Dietary Guideline?

A. maintain healthy body weight.
B. choose a diet low in sugar.
C. choose a diet low in sodium.
D. choose a diet low in starch.

_D_ 6.   The RDA stands for:

A. recommended daily allowance.
B. required dietary allowance.
C. required daily allowance.
D. recommended dietary allowance.

_D_ 7.   The basic watch words of nutrition are?

A. variety.   C. balance.
B. moderation.   D. all of the above.

_D_ 8.   Labeling laws require that ingredients in food products be listed on the container in descending order of their:

A. kcalories.   C. nutrient density.
B. cost.   D. weight.

_A_ 9.   An estimated safe and adequate daily dietary allowance:

A. is set for some nutrients instead of an RDA.
B. gives a range for the RDA.
C. is used to set the U.S. RDA.
D. reflects weekly needs.

_B_ 10.   The adult U.S. RDA:

A. is designed specifically for Americans, whereas the RDA applies to all people.
B. generally represents the highest nutrient needs in the "adult" RDA category.
C. includes all nutrients.
D. applies to individuals, whereas the RDA applies to groups.

_B_ 11.   Which suggestion would <u>NOT</u> greatly improve the possible nutrient "weaknesses" of the Food Guide Pyramid?

A. use whole grains.   C. eat more broccoli.
B. double milk portions.   D. eat more kidney beans.

_C_ 12.   Dietary Guidelines have been issued primarily to decrease:

A. vitamin E deficiencies in the United States.
B. weaknesses in the Food Guide Pyramid.
C. the incidence of chronic "killer" diseases.
D. weaknesses in the RDA.

_C_ 13.   Food choices in the Exchange System are grouped according to similarities in __________ content.

A. kcalorie, carbohydrate, fat, and vitamin.
B. kcalorie, protein, fat, and vitamin.
C. kcalorie, protein, fat, and carbohydrate.
D. vitamin, mineral, and water.

| __B__ | 14. | Substituting beans and seeds for meats and using whole-grain instead of refined breads and cereals improves the nutrient content of the diet by increasing intake of: |

A. vitamins A, D, and C and calcium.
B. magnesium, vitamin E, vitamin B-6, iron, and zinc.
C. thiamin, calcium, and vitamin D.
D. vitamins B-12 and K, chloride, and magnesium.

| __D__ | 15. | The Food Guide Pyramid provides the full allowance of: |

A. all essential nutrients.
B. all essential nutrients except energy.
C. most of the essential nutrients, along with energy.
D. most of the essential nutrients, except energy, for many people.

| __A__ | 16. | The RDA for energy are based on: |

A. average needs.
B. average needs plus a 30% margin of safety.
C. 90% of average needs.
D. double the minimum requirement.

| __B__ | 17. | When a person exceeds 100% of his RDA, his health will improve. |

A. true.   B. false.

| __D__ | 18. | Besides your doctor, where else might you go for sound nutritional advice? |

A. diet books.   C. restaurant or food service managers.
B. registered nurse.   D. Registered Dietitian.

| __B__ | 19. | A current label on a product that contains fewer than 40 kcalories per serving would denote a _________ food? |

A. altered calorie.   C. low calorie.
B. diet.   D. light.

| __E__ | 20. | Vitamin C will be found in the _________ food group. |

A. Milk, Yogurt, and Cheese
B. Fruits
C. Vegetables
D. Breads, Cereals, Rice, and Pasta
E. both B and C

Chapter 3
Sorting Nutritional Advice: Facts and Fallacies

I.   **Points to consider**

Chapter 3 is designed to allow you to:

1.   Identify sources of nutrition quackery.

2.   Compare the nutritional quality and safety of organically grown foods with those of conventionally grown foods.

3.   Compare and contrast nutritional quality and safety of "health" foods with those of typical foods in a grocery store.

4.   Identify characteristics of meganutrient therapy, herbal therapy, and macrobiotics.

5.   Outline a system to evaluate health and nutrition claims.

6.   Understand the basis of the scientific method as it is used in developing hypotheses and theories in the field of nutrition.

II.   **Word parts**

Complete the following exercise using words in Chapter 3.

Word Part	Meaning	Examples
quack	impostor	__________
organic	pertaining to the body, living	__________
mega	big, great	__________
macro	large, long	__________
syn	with, together	__________
-icide	to kill	__________
herb	leafy plant	__________

III.   **Flash cards**

Cut out and review the flash cards for this chapter in Appendix A.

IV.   Review and synthesis

A.   "Organic food advocates claim these crops offer more nutrition and fewer health hazards than conventionally grown foods. Nutrition scientists find such claims about organically grown produce inherently misleading." Compare and contrast claims made by organic gardeners with the findings of nutrition scientists. (66)

(HINT: Compare their views on pesticides, fertilizers, and nutritional quality of foods.)

<u>Claims of "organic" gardeners</u>   versus   <u>Findings of nutrition scientists</u>

B.   1.   "The practice of commercially adding preservatives and other additives to foods tends to generate more heat than light." List some pros and cons of food additives. (68)

<u>Pros</u>   <u>Cons</u>

2.   "One of three shoppers in health-food stores spend money on dubious nutritional products." Review Table 3-1; have you ever been a victim of any of these claims? Were they beneficial in your opinion? (69)

C.	"A balanced diet following the Food Guide Pyramid provides the nutrients you need to stay healthy. There are some cases, however, when vitamin and mineral supplements should be considered, as recommended by a medical doctor." List four conditions for which supplementation may be recommended as suggested by the American Institute of Nutrition and the American Society for Clinical Nutrition. (74)

a.

b.

c.

d.

D.	1.	"We all need to try to identify fraudulent sales techniques to protect ourselves from deception." In the chapter we caution you to beware of misinformation. List three phrases that should warn you to proceed with caution. (77)

a.

b.

c.

2.	"If you suspect false claims about a product or service, seek answers from reputable sources." The chapter offers some suggestions for reliable sources of nutrition information. Name four below. (83)

a.

b.

c.

d.

E.   1.   "How can freedoms of speech and press harm the consumer and protect the phony food promoter?" Design your own venture to promote a "quack" product or service, then verbally promote the claim to family and friends. Note their reactions. (78)

Did they believe you?

What questions did they ask?

Was there a common characteristic among those who believed you? Why is this important?

2.   "The bias (prejudice) of the subject or the experimenter can easily affect the outcome of an experiment." Based on information in the Nutrition Issue, design a simple double-blind study to test whether high doses of vitamin C cure baldness. (91)

Check your answer on page 42 of this <u>Study Guide</u>.

V. **Applying nutrition to your life**

Is the health food store all it's cracked up to be? Many people believe that health food stores are a better place to buy certain foods and supplements than conventional markets. However, identical product brands are often found in both types of stores. In this assignment you are asked to do a price comparison of foods in a health-food store and those in a conventional market.

1. Go to the local health-food store and pick six food items that you think would be sold at a conventional market. Pick plain items like raisins, brown rice, honey, and kidney beans. Also note the type of supplements available in health-food stores. Does it surprise you that people feel the need to purchase and use many of these products?

2. Record the price and weight of the six food items.

3. Calculate the price per pound or ounce.
    Example: a 12-ounce jar of honey costs $3.48.
    $3.48 / 12 ounces = $.29 per ounce

4. Find the same items in a conventional supermarket.

5. Do steps 2 and 3 above for these products.

6. Compare these products based on price per amount (as in pound or ounce).

7. Are the prices consistently higher at the health-food store than at the conventional market? If so, do you see any reason why the products should be more expensive?

Fill in the blanks using the words listed at the end of this summary.

Though capable of causing bodily harm, __________ hits hardest in dollars and cents. Abandoning medical therapy for quack cures may result in needless __________ distress.

__________ and natural foods provide alternatives to foods containing artificial ingredients and __________, and to foods grown with chemical fertilizers and __________. But the overall health and nutritional benefits are few, if any.

Quacks often suggest that the average diet lacks __________ and minerals and so should be supplemented with these products. Choosing whole grains, fruits, and vegetables and other selections from the __________ provides excellent nutrition. An excess of certain vitamins and minerals, such as vitamins A and D and the minerals iron and copper, can cause __________.

__________ remedies and megadose vitamin and mineral therapies seldom help, provide no extra energy and may be __________.

Consumers feeling short changed by conventional health care provide a large and willing market for those promoting questionable and dangerous nutritional advice. Before "buying" into alternative health products or suggestions, check for supporting evidence and __________. If in doubt, check with a __________ or Registered Dietitian.

Any new recommendation for changes in diet habits should be evaluated by using __________ that can either support or refute the recommendation. The health of nutrition science is fostered by a __________ that does not accept a hypothesis as "fact" until manifest proof is available. Until that point, __________ and __________ for a nutrient should be the watchwords. However, if data or evidence from many experiments support a hypothesis, it becomes so generally accepted by scientists that it can be called a __________.

Use the following words to complete the summary

additives	organically grown	reputable credentials
dangerous	pesticides	rigorous experiments
Food Guide Pyramid	physician	skeptical mind
harm	physical	theory
herbal	quackery	variety
moderation		vitamins

Check your answers using the summary for Chapter 3 in your textbook and page 42 for the final five answers.

VII.   Practice examination

Cover the answers on your initial attempt.

__A__   1.   Americans spend over _____________ dollars a year on quackery.

        A. 3 billion   C. 25 billion
        B. 70 billion   D. 125 billion

__B__   2.   One group which seems particularly vulnerable to quackery is:

        A. mothers.   C. teenagers.
        B. elderly persons.   D. religious persons.

__A__   3.   Who is ultimately responsible for protecting you from false advertising and misleading health claims?

        A. yourself   C. government
        B. doctors   D. radio, television, and newspaper executives

__B__   4.   Organically grown foods are much safer and provide better nutrient quality than conventionally grown foods.

        A. True   B. False

__B__   5.   Which of the following terms typically would not be used to define the word natural?

        A. minimal processing   C. no additives
        B. recycled   D. no artificial ingredients

__D__   6.   Grains such as wheat and rice provide many nutrients. However, there is one part of the grain that is indigestible and must be stripped away. This is known as the:

        A. gum.   C. bran.
        B. starch.   D. hull.

__D__   7.   Which of the following functions is an additive capable of doing?

        A. preventing off flavors   C. retaining food crispness
        B. enhancing nutrient value   D. all of the above

__A__   8.   Which of the following is a typical characteristic of foods in a health food store?

        A. they cost more.   C. the food contains extra nutrients.
        B. these are foods we   D. the food is always fresh.
            need that cannot be
            found elsewhere.

__B__   9.   It is a proven fact that stress raises vitamin needs.

        A. True.   B. False.

__B__   10.   The terms snakeroot, sarsaparilla, cumin, and caraway are all names of:

        A. pesticides.   C. sources of meganutrients.
        B. herb products.   D. synthetic drugs.

__D__   11.   Which of the following most accurately defines herbs?

        A. contain magical properties
        B. useful medicines
        C. completely safe
        D. they necessitate caution and medical guidance with use

<u> C </u>   12.   Macrobiotics, originated by philosopher George Ohsawa, originally emphasized a diet rich in:

A. foods of animal origin.   C. vegetables and brown rice.
B. whole grain and soybean products.   D. nuts and seeds.

<u> B </u>   13.   In former and current macrobiotic diets, one important type of food that is often missing is:

A. whole grains.   C. vegetables.
B. milk products.   D. sweets.

<u> D </u>   14.   The American Association of Nutrition Consultants and the International Academy of Nutrition Consultants both:

A. are highly rated professional organizations of nutrition science.
B. give advance training in nutrition consulting.
C. are elite groups of nutrition experts.
D. are places where one can purchase degrees.

<u> D </u>   15.   Which of the following has (have) been known to provide misleading nutritional information:

A. Nutritional Health Federation.
B. pharmacists.
C. health food stores.
D. all of the above.

Match the following hucksters with their theory.

A.   James Caleb Jackson   D. Adele Davis
B.   Bernarr MacFadden   E. Carlton Fredericks
C.   Horace Fletcher   F. Lendon H. Smith

<u> A </u>   16.   Placed rock-hard bits of baked wheat in water to soften and called it granola.

<u> B </u>   17.   Believed that fasting would cure some 30 diseases and that drinking a half gallon of water each morning would strengthen the heart and prevent constipation.

<u> E </u>   18.   Though he had no nutrition and health science training, he often diagnosed patients and prescribed vitamins to remove the aches and pains of illness.

<u> D </u>   19.   Proposed that people should take vitamins and supplements and eat organic fruit and vegetables, wheat germ, raw milk, stone ground 100% whole-grain bread or cereal and other "health" food products.

<u> C </u>   20.   Believing that large chunks of food interfered with digestion, he advocated chewing until food "swallowed itself".

<u> F </u>   21.   Claimed that allergies, hyperactivity, and a variety of other ailments in children result from enzyme disturbances that dietary changes can help.

<u> A </u>   22.   A safe standard of one's RDA is to meet a least 70%. Keep in mind, however, some nutrients are potentially toxic at high doses. So it is best not to exceed _________ of the RDA unless under medical supervision.

A. 150%   C. 500%
B. 200%   D. 1000%

<u> A </u>   23.   Epidemiological studies yield nutrition information through:

A. correlations of diets with disease in certain populations.
B. study of archaeological findings.
C. laboratory experiments.
D. chemical analysis of foods.

41

| __B__ | 24. | When scientists observe occurrences that cannot be explained, they attempt to formulate questions that may provide possible explanations for the phenomena. Another name for these questions are: |

A. theories.   C. experiments.
B. hypertension.   D. diabetes.

| __E__ | 25. | Quackery can significantly harm or kill its victims by: |

A. promoting unsafe or hazardous products.
B. delaying effective treatment for serious conditions.
C. abandoning effective treatment.
D. impoverishment. Victims are harmed economically.
E. A, B, and C.

Answers to selected questions

IV. E. 2.   Double-blind study: Find 20 bald men. Give 10 men a high dose of vitamin C each day for a month, while the other 10 men receive a placebo ("fake medicine"). Neither the subjects nor you can know who receives which treatment. Your friend holds the code and only divulges it after the experiment ends and any new hair growth is documented.

VI.   rigorous experiments; skeptical mind; variety; moderation; theory

---

Chapter 4
The Human Body: A Nutrition Perspective

I.   **Points to consider**

Chapter 4 is designed to allow you to:

1.   Outline the organs used in digestion and absorption.

2.   Describe the function of each organ used in the digestive process and the flow of the process.

3.   Name the enzyme classes that act on each nutrient group.

4.   Describe the mechanisms used for food absorption into the body.

5.   Outline the role of the heart, kidneys, nerves, muscles, hormones, and hormone-like factors in digestion and absorption.

6.   Identify some conditions that result when digestive processes are hampered.

II.   **Word parts**

Complete the following exercise using words in Chapter 4.

Word part	Meaning	Examples
gastr	stomach	__________
col	colon	__________
zym	ferment	__________
aut	self	__________
phag	eat	__________
hepat	liver	__________
peps	digest	__________
ase	enzyme	__________

III.   **Flash cards**

Cut out and review the flash cards for this chapter in Appendix A.

A.   1.   "Often two or more tissues combine to form more complex organs." Briefly define the
              following terms. (96)

              a.   cell

              b.   tissue

              c.   organ

              d.   organ system (e.g. bone)

       2.   "As the embryo forms, different parts of the DNA become active." Describe how DNA
              allows for the development of different cells, and in doing so, different organ systems.
              (97)

B.   Describe the roles the following organism systems play in the nutritional processes and overall
       health of the body.

              a.   circulatory system

              b.   hormonal systems

              c.   nervous system

              d.   excretory system

              e.   storage systems (e.g. adipose cells)

              f.   immune system

C.	"The hormone cholecystokinin (CCK) controls the release of enzymes--like lipase--from the pancreas." Complete the descriptions of the hormones that regulate the digestive tract. (99)

Hormone	Origin	Stimulus to secretion	Action
gastrin		food and other substances in the stomach, especially proteins, caffeine, spices, and alcohol; nerve input	
	upper small intestine		inhibits secretion of stomach acid and enzymes; reduces stomach motility
cholecystokinin		food, especially fat and protein in the upper small intestine	
secretin			causes secretion of thin, bicarbonate-rich pancreatic juice; reduces stomach contractions

D.   "Enzymes enhance digestion by making chemical reactions more likely to happen." Complete this summary of digestive enzymes. (104)

Secretion origin	Enzyme	Substrate	Major end products
1. salivary glands	salivary amylase	starch, glycogen	maltose
2. stomach glands	pepsin	_________	smaller proteins
3. _____________	_____________	proteins	_____________
	chymotrypsin	_________	peptides
	_____________	starch	maltose
	lipase	_________	monoglycerides, free fatty acids
4. intestinal wall	peptidase	peptides	_______, _______
	_____________	maltose	_____________
	sucrase	_________	glucose, _________
	_____________	lactose	_________, _______

E.   "Fluids and particles leaving the villi in the intestine drain into two different circulation systems." Classify each term in the box with the expected transport system. (97)

Portal vein	Lymphatic vessels
_____________	_____________
_____________	_____________
_____________	
_____________	
_____________	

alcohol
amino acids
fat-soluble vitamins
minerals
monosaccharides
triglycerides
  (long-chain)
water-soluble vitamins

Check your answers on page 54 in this <u>Study Guide</u>.

F.   "Specialized enzymes made by the absorptive cells of the small intestine then break down the many dietary sugars." Malabsorption of lactose, as you will further research in Chapter 5, may cause bloating, diarrhea, flatus, and abdominal discomfort. Why? (103)

G.   1.   "In the small intestine, absorption occurs by various processes." What is active absorption? (107)

Why is it necessary for glucose?

2.   Describe the two other main types of absorption.

H.   "The presence of feces in the rectum stimulates elimination." What are two functions of the large intestine? (108)

a.

b.

I.   "A person who is prone to developing ulcers should not smoke." Provide some dietary and other practical advice for people who suffer from the following disorders: (117)

      a.   ulcers

      b.   heartburn

      c.   constipation

      d.   hemorrhoids

     Applying nutrition to your life

"The gastrointestinal tract is also known as the alimentary canal." Label each part indicated in the figure using the following terms, and briefly describe each part's role, if any, in digestion and absorption. Check your answers using Figures 4-3, 4-5, and page 101 in your textbook.

---

pancreas, anus, trachea, salivary glands, appendix, mouth, esophagus, large intestine (colon), liver, rectum, stomach, small intestine, epiglottis, gallbladder, pyloric sphincter, common bile duct

---

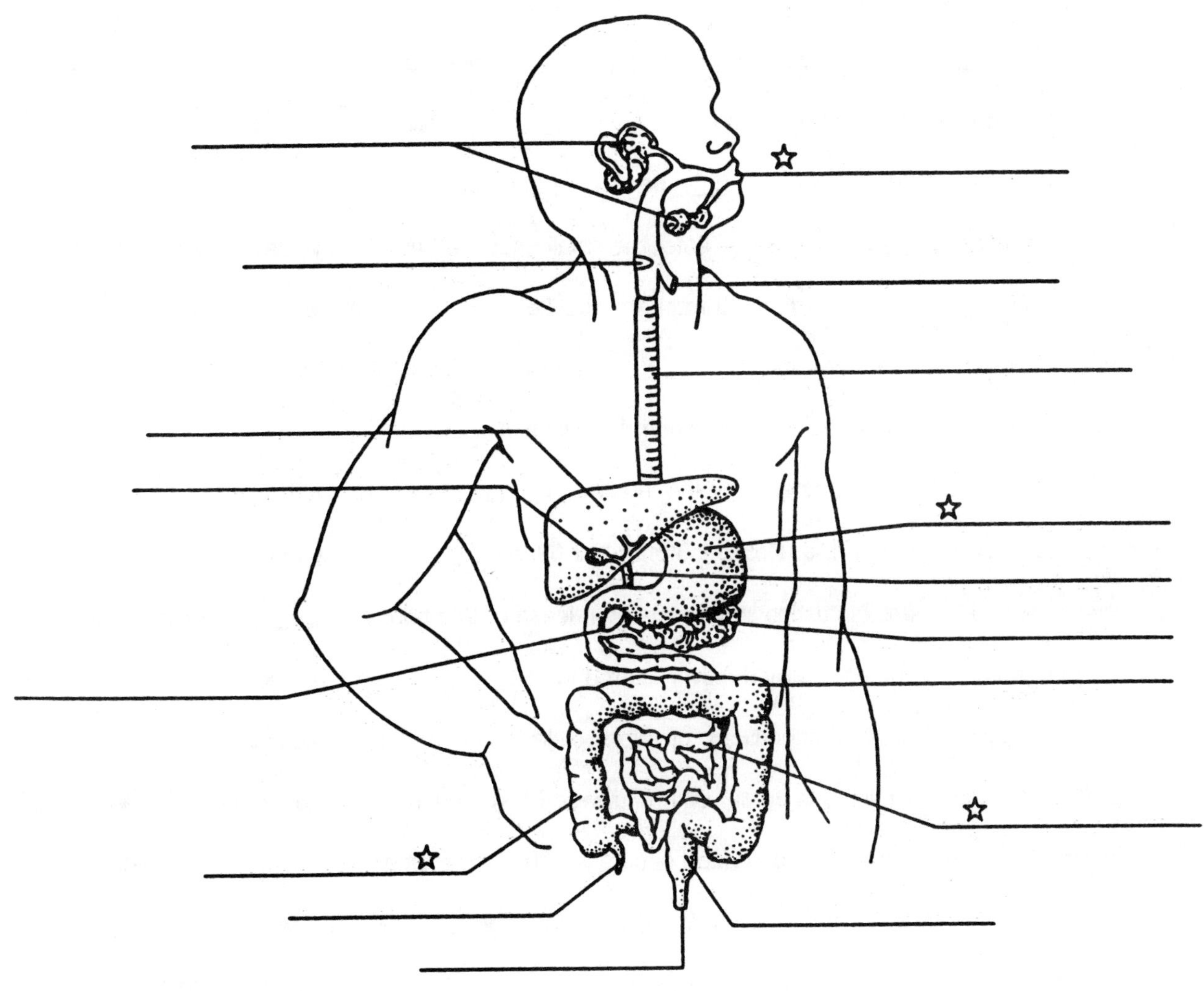

49

Fill in the blanks using the words listed at the end of this summary.

The __________ is the basic building block of body tissues. __________ is the blueprint found in all cells. It determines the cell type as it is used to produce specific __________ and __________ for each type of cell. Blood travels the __________, in which oxygen is picked up by the lungs. The systemic circuit delivers essential nutrients, energy, __________, and water to all body cells. Nutrients and wastes are exchanged between the blood and the cell across the __________. Water-soluble compounds in the __________ enter the __________ and travel to the liver. Fat-soluble compounds enter into the __________, which eventually connects to the __________.

The ____________ consists of the mouth, __________, stomach, __________, large intestine (colon), rectum, and anus. Most digestion and __________ of nutrients occurs in the small intestine. The __________, gallbladder, and __________ participate in digestion and absorption. Products from these organs -- like __________ and bile -- enter the small intestine and play important roles in digesting protein, fat, and __________. Along the GI tract are ringlike __________ that control the flow of foodstuffs. Muscular contractions, called __________, propel the foodstuffs down the GI tract. A variety of nerves, hormones and other substances, control the process.

Digestive enzymes are secreted by the mouth, __________, and wall of the __________ intestine and pancreas. Pancreatic enzyme release is controlled by the __________ cholecystokinin (CCK). The presence of food in the small intestine stimulates the release of this hormone. __________ needed for __________ digestion is synthesized by the liver, stored in the __________, and released in digestion. The major absorptive sites consist of fingerlike projections called villi in the small intestine. __________ cover the villi. Thus the intestinal lining is continually renewed. Most digestion and absorption occurs in the small intestine. Little digestion and absorption occurs in either the stomach or __________ intestine. Some __________ are digested in the stomach. Some plant fibers are digested by the __________ present in the __________. Final water and mineral absorption takes place in the large intestine. The presence of __________ in the __________ provides a strong impetus for elimination.

A person who is prone to developing ulcers should not _______________. Minimizing the use of

_____________ also is important because of its resulting irritation to the stomach. This combination of

therapies, along with the use of antacids and other anti-acid medications, has revolutionized ulcer

therapy. An important dietary measure for avoiding heartburn is to eat _________ meals low in fat.

Meals containing much fat remain in the stomach longer and create pressure in the stomach that can

force stomach _________ into the esophagus.

Use the following words to complete the summary

absorption	fat	proteins
absorptive cells	feces	portal vein
acid	fluid	pulmonary circuit
aspirin	gallbladder	rectum
bacteria	gastrointestinal	small
bile	(GI) tract	smaller
bloodstream	hormone	small intestine
carbohydrates	large	smoke
cell	large intestine	stomach
cell membrane	liver	structures
chemicals	lymphatic system	triglycerides
DNA	oxygen	valves (sphincters)
enzymes	pancreas	villi
esophagus	peristalsis	

Check your answers using the summary for Chapter 4 in your textbook and page 54 of this <u>Study Guide</u>
for the last four answers.

Cover the answers on your initial attempt.

__B__   1.   The best treatment for an ulcer is the milk and cream therapy.

A. True   B. False

__C__   2.   The liver is the first stop for most absorbed nutrients because it:

A. lies so close to the intestine.
B. controls blood flow to the heart.
C. is the end point for the portal vein.
D. must respond by making the correct amount of insulin.

__C__   3.   The major site for fluid absorption in the gastrointestinal tract is the:

A. esophagus.   C. small intestine.
B. stomach.   D. colon.

__D__   4.   The gnawing pain in the upper chest that is caused by acid flowing back into the esophagus from the stomach is termed:

A. lactose intolerance.   C. hemorrhoids.
B. ulcer.   D. heartburn.

__C__   5.   The function of mucus in the stomach is to:

A. neutralize stomach acid.
B. activate pepsinogen to form pepsin.
C. protect stomach cells from autodigestion.
D. emulsify fats.

__D__   6.   The pyloric sphincter:

A. prevents the contents of the intestine from backing up into the stomach.
B. secretes acid into the stomach.
C. holds the food in the stomach long enough for it to be thoroughly mixed and liquefied.
D. A and C.

__C__   7.   A sensible idea for preventing constipation is to:

A. use a laxative when needed.
B. cut down on water intake.
C. include more high-fiber foods in the diet.
D. include fewer high-fiber foods in the diet.

__C__   8.   The lining of the gastrointestinal tract is replaced completely about every:

A. 12 hours.   C. 2 to 5 days.
B. 1 day.   D. 2 weeks.

__A__   9.   Cholecystokinin is:

A. formed in the duodenum and stimulates gallbladder and pancreatic secretions.
B. part of the bile.
C. formed in the stomach and causes gastric juice to be secreted.
D. an outdated name for secretin.

_C_   10.   Nutrients that enter the lymph for absorption are:

A. ascorbic acid, minerals, amino acids, and cholesterol.
B. short-chain fatty acids, triglycerides, and cholesterol.
C. long-chain fatty acids, triglycerides, and vitamin A.
D. minerals, short-chain fatty acids, and carotene.

_D_   11.   Much of the digestion that occurs in the large intestine is caused by:

A. lipase.   C. saliva.
B. pepsin.   D. bacteria.

<u>Match the following:</u>

_C_	12.	peristalsis	A.	Acts as a lubricant and protein for stomach cells.
_I_	13.	sphincter	B.	This transport system requires that energy be expended by the cell to pump a compound into the cell.
_H_	14.	chyme		
_A_	15.	mucus		
_G_	16.	tissue	C.	Muscle contractions of the gut.
_E_	17.	epiglottis	D.	Molecules cross cell membranes without use of carrier molecules or energy expenditure.
_F_	18.	colon		
_B_	19.	active absorption	E.	Closes off the trachea during swallowing to prevent food from entering the lungs.
_E_	20.	passive diffusion	F.	Reabsorbs water from undigested food and waste materials.
			G.	A group of cells designed to perform a specific function.
			H.	A mixture of stomach secretions and partially digested foods.
			I.	A muscular valve that controls flow of food stuff.

_B_   21.   The portal vein:

A. carries blood from the lungs to the heart.
B. collects blood from the intestinal capillary bed and carries it to the liver.
C. delivers fat and soluble compounds to the lymphatic system.
D. is also known as the alimentary canal.

_D_   22.   Short-term storage of carbohydrate occurs:

A. in the intestinal mucosa.
B. when the skin is exposed to the sun.
C. as amino acid reserves in the bloodstream.
D. in the muscle and liver.

_C_   23.   Bile is formed in the:

A. pancreas.   C. liver.
B. walls of the small intestine.   D. gallbladder.

_A_   24.   Digestion begins in the:

A. mouth.   C. small intestine.
B. stomach.   D. pancreas.

_D_   25.   The action of pancreatic lipase digests triglycerides and phospholipids to produce:

A. diglycerides.   C. fatty acids.
B. monoglycerides.   D. both B and C.

IV. D.   portal vein   alcohol, amino acids, minerals, monosaccharides, water-soluble vitamins

lymphatic vessels   fat-soluble vitamins, triglycerides (long-chain)

VI.   smoke; aspirin; smaller; acid.

Chapter 5
Carbohydrates: Sugars, Starches and Dietary Fibers

I. **Points to consider**

Chapter 5 is designed to allow you to:

1. Relate the major carbohydrates: monosaccharides, disaccharides, and polysaccharides, and dietary fiber in terms of their basic structures and food sources.

2. List the functions of carbohydrate in the body and the problems that result from not eating enough.

3. Describe the regulation of one's blood glucose level and the nutrients that can become blood glucose.

4. Outline the effects of dietary fiber on the body.

5. List guidelines for carbohydrate intake.

6. Describe food sources of carbohydrate and list some alternate sweeteners.

7. Identify the consequences of lactose intolerance and diabetes, and appropriate dietary measures to take to reduce these health problems.

II. **Word parts**

Complete the following exercise using words in Chapter 5.

Word part	Meaning	Examples
mono	one	_____________
poly	many	_____________
ose	sugar	_____________
glyc	glucose	_____________
hyper	over, above	_____________
hypo	under	_____________
sacchar	sugar	_____________

III.   **Flash cards**

Cut out and review the flash cards for this chapter in Appendix A.

IV.   **Review and synthesis**

A.   "In digestion, starches, also known as complex carbohydrates, are transformed into the single
sugar glucose." Describe the digestion of a breakfast, consisting of a glass of grape juice, a
slice of toast with jelly, and a bowl of cereal and milk by indicating the part of the digestive tract
where each of the following occur. (123)

1. ______   The disaccharides, sucrose (in the jelly) and lactose (in the milk), are broken
down by enzymes into their respective monosaccharides.

2. ______   Starch (in the bread and cereal) is broken down by the enzyme salivary
amylase.

3. ______   Starch, and its partial breakdown products, are broken down to maltose by the
enzyme pancreatic amylase.

4. ______   Salivary amylase is inactivated by strong acid. The digestion of starch is then
temporarily halted.

5. ______   Absorption of glucose, fructose (from the grape juice), and galactose (from the
milk sugar) takes place.

B.   1.   "The main function of glucose is to supply energy for the body. Certain tissues in the
body, such as red blood cells, can use only this and other simple carbohydrate forms
for energy." Describe briefly three functions of carbohydrates. (126)

a.

b.

c.

2.   "Under normal circumstances, a person's blood glucose level is regulated within a very
narrow range." The hormones that regulate blood glucose levels include: (127)

a.

b.

c.

Briefly note the effects of each on blood sugar levels.

3. "On the tip of the tongue are receptors for tasting sweetness." Rank these sugars in order of sweetness. (128)

maltose, sucrose, glucose, fructose, sorbitol

How does the sweetness of aspartame compare to these sugars?

4. "If you don't eat enough carbohydrate your body is forced to make glucose from other nutrients." Briefly describe what medical problems are associated with a low-carbohydrate diet. (Hint: what happens to protein and other body constituents when carbohydrates cannot be used as an energy source?) (128)

a.

b.

C. 1. "Dietary fiber is not a single substance, but actually a group of substances with similar characteristics." Complete this table on the classification of dietary fibers. (131)

Type	Component	Examples	Physiological effects	Major food sources
Insoluble				
Noncarbohydrate	______	______	Uncertain	All plants
Carbohydrate	Cellulose	______	Increases fecal bulk	______
	______	Brown rice	Decreases transit time	Wheat, ______, ______, ______
Soluble				
Carbohydrate	______, gums, ______	Apples, ______, ______, Carrots, barley, ______, ______	Delays gastric emptying; slows glucose absorption; ______	______, oat products, ______

2.   "When enough fiber is consumed, its water-retaining property helps enlarge and soften the stool, easing elimination." List two potential benefits of fiber in the diet. (132)

    a.

    b.

D.   1.   "Most of these sugars are added to foods and beverages." Provide some suggestions for lowering sugar intake that seem reasonable to you. (141)

<u>Instead of:</u>   <u>Try:</u>

Sweet desserts

____

Soda or powdered drink mixes

____

Sugar-coated cereals

____

Candy

____

Canned fruit in heavy syrup

____

Sweet rolls or doughnuts

____

2.	Use Appendix A in your textbook or your computer software to predict the kcalories and carbohydrate content in the following one-day diet.

Foods	Kcalories	Carbohydrate (grams)
Breakfast		
3/4 cup Cheerios cereal		
1 cup 2% milk		
1/2 cup orange juice		
Lunch		
3 ounces broiled hamburger		
1 hamburger bun		
1 ounce cheddar cheese		
1 tablespoon mustard		
1 cup 2% milk		
1 apple		
Dinner		
3 ounces broiled chicken		
1/3 cup rice		
1/2 cup broccoli		
1 teaspoon margarine		
TOTALS:	_____ kcalories	_____ grams of carbohydrate

What percentage of kcalories does carbohydrate contribute to this diet? _________ %

See page 64 of this <u>Study Guide</u> to check your numerical answers.

E.	"Much lactose is lost when milk is made into cheese." Provide four tips to a person with lactose intolerance in both reducing symptoms and having a healthy diet. (125)

    a.

    b.

    c.

    d.

F.   "Aspartame yields 4 kcalories per gram but little need be used in foods since it is 200 times sweeter than sucrose." Briefly describe the current uses and controversies surrounding the use of the following alternate sweeteners. (143)

    a.   aspartame (NutraSweet)

    b.   saccharin

    c.   acesulfame K (Sunette)

V.   **Applying nutrition to your life**

"Although a desirable level of sugar intake has not yet been set, less than 10%-15% of total kcalorie intake is considered a recommended level." First pick a weekend or weekday that would reflect a day as your greatest consumption of sugar (sweet foods). Write down all the sugared (sweet) foods you ate for that day. Look up the number of teaspoons of sugar in these foods in Table 5-5. Record this information in the table below.

<u>Sugars and sweet foods</u>   <u>Teaspoons of sugar</u>

_______________ total teaspoons

How many teaspoons of sugar did you eat?

Put an X on the scale below where your sugar consumption rates:

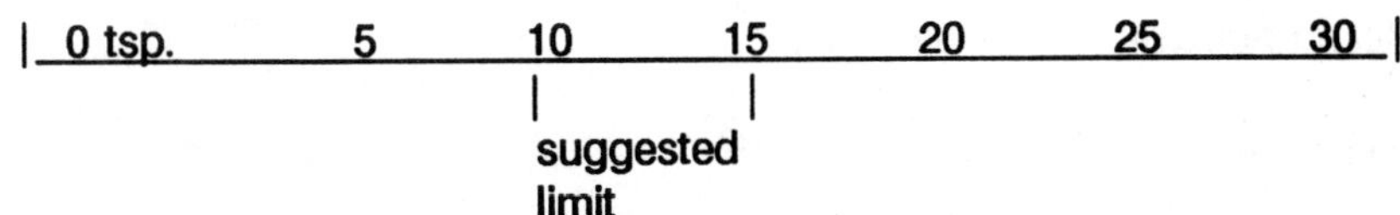

Did you exceed 10-15 teaspoons? How could you change your intake to reduce your sugar consumption?

Fill in the blanks using the words listed at the end of this summary.

The monosaccharides in our diet include glucose, __________, and __________. Once absorbed by the small intestine and passed to the liver, these mostly leave as __________. The major disaccharides in nutrition are __________ (glucose plus fructose), __________ (glucose plus glucose), and __________ (glucose plus galactose). These are digested to form their __________. The major polysaccharides in our diet contain __________ glucose units linked together. A straight-chained form is __________, and __________ is an animal starch and acts as a storage form of carbohydrate in the liver.

Some __________ digestion occurs in the mouth. In the __________ carbohydrate digestion is finished. Some plant fibers are digested by the __________ present in the colon.

Lactose is the sugar found in __________. __________ results when cells of the intestinal wall do not make sufficient __________, the enzyme necessary to digest lactose. Undigested lactose travels to the __________, resulting in symptoms such as abdominal gas, pain and __________. Some people with lactose intolerance can tolerate cheeses, yogurt, and small amounts of milk, though tolerance to __________ as a whole is very individualistic.

The carbohydrates in our diet provide __________, protect against the needless metabolism of protein to supply glucose for the body's needs, prevent ketosis, and provide __________ to foods. Simple carbohydrates can be metabolized to __________ by bacteria on teeth. The acid can erode the tooth surfaces leading to __________. The dietary fibers include __________, hemicelluloses, pectins, __________, mucilages, and lignins. These can provide mass to the __________, in turn easing __________.

There is no __________ for carbohydrate. An intake of 50 to 100 grams per day should prevent __________. About __________ of total kcalories is recommended. If inadequate carbohydrate intake continues for weeks at a time, the price is a loss of __________ protein, ketosis, and general weakness of the body. Diets high in __________ carbohydrates are encouraged today to replace diets high in

___________. Foods to emphasize are potatoes, grains, pastas, and vegetables. Sugar intake should be limited to ___________ of kcalories.

Diabetes mellitus is characterized by ___________ blood glucose levels. Treatments for the disease can include a regulated carbohydrate/protein/fat consumption, use of insulin, weight loss, regular ___________, and oral hypoglycemic agents, depending on the type of diabetes. True ___________ is rare. ___________ at every meal is a recommended therapy.

Use the following words to complete the summary

acid	energy	high	protein
amylose	elimination	hypoglycemia	RDA
bacteria	fat	ketosis	small intestine
body	feces	lactase	starch
cellulose	flavor and	lactose	sucrose
colon	sweetness	maltose	10%
complex	fructose	milk	55%
dairy products	galactose	monosaccharide	
dental caries	glucose	multiple	
diarrhea	glycogen	physical activity	
	gums		

Check your answers using the summary for Chapter 5 in your textbook and the next page of this <u>Study Guide</u> for the last four answers.

IV. D. 2. approximate kcalories = 80 + 120 + 60 + 225 + 160 + 100 + 0 + 120 + 60 + 165+ 80 + 25 + 45 = <u>1260 kcalories</u>

carbohydrate = 15 + 12 + 15 + 0 + 30 + 0 + 0 + 12 + 15 + 0 + 15 + 5 + 0 = <u>119 grams of carbohydrate</u>

$$((119 \times 4) / 1260) \times 100 = 38\% \text{ kcals as carbohydrates}$$

VI. high; physical activity; hypoglycemia; protein

VII. Practice examination

Cover the answers on your initial attempt.

__B__ 1. Cellulose, hemicelluloses, and lignins are fibers found in:

A. ripe fruits.
B. plant walls, skins, peels, and bran layers of grains.
C. pectin.
D. food additives such as guar gum.

__C__ 2. In calculating the fiber content of your diet, the best value to use is the:

A. percentage of kcalories from carbohydrates.
B. total grams of carbohydrates.
C. dietary fiber value.
D. crude fiber value.

__C__ 3. It is recommended that about ______ of your total kcalorie intake come from carbohydrates.

A. 10%   C. 55%
B. 30%   D. 70%

__A__ 4. Allen consumed 3200 kcalories yesterday containing 100 grams of carbohydrate. What percentage of his kcalories came from the carbohydrates?

A. 12%   C. 50%
B. 25%   D. 75%

__D__ 5. A high fiber diet:

A. is encouraged by a meat and potatoes menu.
B. is good insurance against diarrhea.
C. causes diverticulosis.
D. reduces transit time.

__A__ 6. Which of the following is another name for glucose?

A. dextrose.   C. fruit sugar.
B. disaccharide.   D. all of the above.

| C | 7. | The primary source of carbohydrates in the diet comes from which of the following group of foods? |

    A. milk and milk products.
    B. breads, cereals, and grain products.
    C. fruits and vegetables.
    D. meat, fish, poultry, and beans.

B   8.   The form of diabetes that often begins in late childhood and is characterized by the pancreas' inability to make insulin is called:

    A. hypoglycemla.   C. noninsulin dependent diabetes.
    B. insulin-dependent diabetes.   D. hyperglycemia.

For questions 9 through 12 identify the following carbohydrates:

D   9.   animal starch   A. sucrose

B   10.   monosaccharide   B. glucose

C   11.   plant starch   C. amylose

A   12.   disaccharide   D. glycogen

B   13.   Which of the following hormones lowers blood glucose levels?

    A. glucagon.   C. epinephrine.
    B. insulin.   D. cortisol.

D   14.   The RDA for carbohydrates is:

    A. 44 grams.   C. 50 to 55 milligrams.
    B. 800 RE   D. nonexistent; there is no RDA for carbohydrates.

C   15.   Aspartame:

    A. is stable at high temperatures.
    B. may cause cancer.
    C. contains about 4 kcalories per gram.
    D. is a carbohydrate.

D   16.   Polysaccharides are made of:

    A. one molecule of sugar.
    B. two monosaccharides linked together.
    C. three monosaccharides linked together.
    D. many monosaccharides linked together.

A   17.   What is the major problem associated with a diet high in simple sugar?

    A. lack of fiber   C. diabetes
    B. hyperglycemia   D. dental caries

B   18.   Dental caries are caused by:

    A. sugar in the mouth eroding the tooth enamel.
    B. acids produced by bacteria as they metabolize carbohydrates.
    C. bacteria directly digesting tooth enamel.
    D. saliva in the mouth.

<u>B</u>   19.   When sucrose is digested it yields:

A. two maltose units.
B. glucose and fructose.
C. glucose and galactose.
D. fructose and galactose.

<u>D</u>   20.   Sucrose is not as sweet as:

A. starch.   C. galactose.
B. maltose.   D. fructose.

<u>B</u>   21.   To metabolize fats adequately, the diet should contain _______ grams of carbohydrates.

A. 20 to 25   C. 100 to 200
B. 50 to 100   D. 200 to 300

<u>D</u>   22.   The best type of fiber to eat for reducing constipation is:

A. glycogen.   C. soluble fiber.
B. crude fiber.   D. insoluble fiber.

<u>B</u>   23.   The chief function of carbohydrates we eat is to:

A. maintain body fat.
B. provide energy.
C. provide essential amino acids.
D. transport vitamin A.

<u>C</u>   24.   A high-carbohydrate diet:

A. is necessarily fattening.
B. causes ketosis.
C. is protein-sparing.
D. forces glucose production from protein.

<u>D</u>   25.   The symptoms of lactose intolerance are mainly caused by eventual lactose breakdown by bacteria in the:

A. mouth.   C. small intestine.
B. stomach.   D. large intestine (colon).

Chapter 6
Lipids: Fats and Oils

I.   **Points to consider**

Chapter 6 is designed to allow you to:

1.   List four classes of fats and their importance for nutritional health.

2.   Differentiate between monoglycerides, diglycerides, and triglycerides.

3.   Differentiate between saturated, monounsaturated, and polyunsaturated fatty acids in terms of structure and food sources.

4.   Name the essential fatty acids and explain why they are called "essential".

5.   Name the classes of lipoproteins and classify them according to their functions.

6.   Discuss the implications of fat, including the omega-3 fatty acids, with respect to coronary heart disease.

7.   Characterize signs and symptoms of heart disease and highlight some known risk factors.

8.   Identify hidden fat in foods and name available fat replacements.

II.   **Word parts**

Complete the following exercise using words in Chapter 6.

Word Part	Meaning	Examples
lip	lipid, fat	__________
phos	phosphorus	__________
philic	loving, affinity for	__________
phobic	fear	__________
tri	three	__________
hydro	water	__________

III.   **Flash cards**

Cut out and review the flash cards for this chapter in Appendix A.

IV.   **Review and synthesis**

A.   "Once dietary fat is digested and absorbed into the small intestine's cells, triglycerides are reformed." To review important concepts about lipid digestion, complete the following exercise. (166)

1.   Fat digestion primarily occurs in the ___________.

2.   Describe the role of bile in the digestion of fat.

3.   Three end products of fat digestion are:

a.

b.

c.

4.   "After digestion and then absorption into the cells of the small intestine, fat is transported throughout the body in the form of _________." The four major classes and functions of this and other lipoprotein compounds are: (168)

a.

b.

c.

d.

B. 1. "Fats are a diverse group of chemical compounds, but they share one main characteristic: they do not dissolve in water." Name three types of fats, excluding fatty acids. (156)

a.

b.

c.

Briefly note the basic function of each.

The largest portion of fat in the food supply and in your body is in the form

of________________________. (161)

A monoglyceride contains glycerol and how many fatty acids? ________ (161)

A saturated fatty acid contains how many C=C double bonds? ________ (156)

A polyunsaturated fatty acid contains how many C=C double

bonds? __________ (156)

2. "A shorter chain length overrides the effect of saturation." The physical properties of a fat are determined by what two chemical characteristics? (159)

a.

b.

How do these characteristics explain the properties of coconut oil?

3. "To solidify vegetable oils for this and other uses into shortenings and margarines, the polyunsaturated fatty acids must become more saturated." Name this process and briefly explain how it occurs. Then name two foods you eat that contain these types of fats. (160)

C. 1. "Alpha-linolenic acid is a major omega-3 fatty acid in foods; linoleic acid is the major omega-6 fatty acid." Provide one example to differentiate between the structures and the effects of products made from omega-3 and omega-6 fatty acids. (158)

D. 1. "When we store fats in fat cells, we store little else."
Some functions of fat in the body are: (162)

a.

b.

c.

2. The essential fatty acids are: (156)

a.

b.

E. 1. "For foods in general, the highest nutrient density for fat is found in salad oil, butter, margarine, and mayonnaise; all contain about 100% of kcalories as fat." First rank the foods in fat content from 1 to 10, with 1 being the lowest in fat. (176) Then use Appendix A in your textbook to determine how many grams of fat are actually in each of the foods below. Adjust serving size, and so fat contribution, so that all choices yield 250 kcalories.

1)	croissant	______	6)	Snickers candy bar	______
2)	fried chicken	______	7)	cheddar cheese	______
3)	egg	______	8)	peanuts (oil roasted)	______
4)	roast beef (lean)	______	9)	green split pea soup	______
5)	white rice	______	10)	Triscuits (crackers)	______

2. "The American Heart Association recommends eating no more than 30% of your total kcalories as fats, using nearly equal amounts of saturated, monounsaturated, and polyunsaturated fatty acids." (174) Calculate the total kcalories, grams of fat, and percentage of fat in the following menu. Use Appendix A in your textbook or computer software to assist you.

	A	B
Foods	kcalories	Fat (grams)
Breakfast		
1 cup 2% milk		
1 egg fried in		
1 teaspoon margarine		
2 ounces ham		
2 slices toast		
2 teaspoons margarine		
Lunch		
2 ounces peanut butter		
1/2 banana		
2 slices bread		
1 cup skim milk		
Dinner		
4 ounces tenderloin steak		
2 tablespoons french dressing		
1/2 cup mixed salad		
1 teaspoon margarine		
2 tablespoons sour cream		
1 small potato		
1/2 cup green beans		
1 teaspoon margarine		
TOTAL	______ kcalories	______ grams of fat

What percentage of kcalories does fat contribute to the previous diet? _____________%

(HINT: column B x 9) x 100/column A)

See page 76 of this <u>Study Guide</u> to check your numerical answers.

F.   1.   "Heart disease is the major killer of Americans." What are three key controllable risk factors for heart disease? (185)

     a.

     b.

     c.

2.   Serum cholesterol levels may be raised by what specific components of the diet? Star the most significant component. (186)

     a.

     b.

3.   Serum cholesterol levels may be lowered by what four specific diet changes? (189-190)

     a.

     b.

     c.

     d.

See page 76 of this <u>Study Guide</u> to check your answers.

G. "For years manufacturers have used starch derivatives to bind water in foods in an attempt to find a substitute that captures the feeling of fat in the mouth." Name three fat replacements. Note how they are made and give an example of a current (or potential) food product each is found in. (178)

<u>Name</u>   <u>How made</u>   <u>Example of food product</u>

a.

b.

c.

V. **Applying nutrition to your life.**

How much fat and saturated fat does the AHA feel is too much for you? To determine this, do some calculations.

First record the kcalorie allowance that is appropriate for you. Use the RDA for a rough guideline, or the amount of kcalories you ate listed on your diet analysis.

       kcalorie allowance _______________________________

Now determine how many kcalories of fat you should eat at this level of kcalories. Take 30% of the figure you wrote in the blank above.

       kcalorie allowance x 0.30 ______________
                             (kcals from fat)

Next, take this figure and divide it by the energy value for fat, 9 kcalories/gram.

       kcalories from fat/9 = __________________ grams

Finally, let's determine the most grams of saturated fat you should eat. Take 10% of your kcalorie allowance, then divide the results by 9. This will give you the number of grams of saturated fat you should not exceed.

      __________________ grams of saturated fat

Consult your diet analysis in Chapter 2 in your textbook to see if your fat intake exceeds these values. If so, name three dietary changes you could make to stay within these guidelines.

a.

b.

c.

VI.   Chapter 6 summary

Fill in the blanks using the words listed at the end of this summary.

Lipids are a group of relatively oxygen-poor compounds that do not dissolve in _______. Saturated fatty acids contain _________ C=C double bond(s); monounsaturated fatty acids contain _________ C=C double bond(s). If the C=C double bonds In the fatty acid begin at the third carbon atom from the methyl end (-CH$_3$), then the fatty acid is an _________ fatty acid. If the double bonds begin at the sixth carbon, it is an _________ fatty acid. Both types of these fatty acids are essential parts of a diet. When cells use omega-3 fatty acids to synthesize hormone-like compounds called _________, the products tend to reduce blood clotting, blood pressure, and inflammatory responses in the body.

Because many fish contain ample amounts of beneficial omega-3 fatty acids, eating fish at least _________ a week is a good dietary practice.

Fats composed of saturated fatty acids tend to be _________ at room temperature; those with polyunsaturated fatty acids are usually _________ at room temperature. _________ is the process of turning C=C double bonds in fatty acids into single bonds. Manufacturers hydrogenate fats to solidify vegetable oils for making shortenings and margarines and to reduce the breakdown of polyunsaturated fatty acids, which leads to less _________. Triglyceride is the major form of _________ in food and in the body.

Besides supplying essential fatty acids to the body, triglycerides supply _________, allow efficient energy storage, _________ and protect the body, transport fat-soluble vitamins, provide _________, and add flavor and texture to foods. Phospholipids are derivatives of triglycerides and form parts of _________, and some act as _________. Cholesterol forms vital compounds for the body, such as hormones, parts of cell membranes, and _________. We eat cholesterol and _________ make it.

In the _________ pancreatic _________ digests triglycerides into small breakdown products. These are absorbed into _________ and mostly resynthesized into _________. These are incorporated into _________ and eventually enter the bloodstream through the _________.

Fats are carried in the bloodstream by lipoproteins: chylomicrons, ______________, low density lipoproteins (LDL), and high density lipoproteins (HDL). An elevated serum __________ level is associated with a high risk of heart disease, as is a low serum __________ level. No RDA exists for fat. One needs about __________ of ________ daily to obtain the needed __________. To lower a high serum cholesterol level, one should mainly try to minimize the intake of __________ fatty acids. Major contributors of fat to our diet include animal foods, __________, and pastries. The fat substitute __________ will allow us to eat some dairy products, such as frozen desserts, without consuming much fat.

Use the following words to complete the summary

absorptive cells	HDL cholesterol	omega-3	solid
bile acids	hydrogenation	omega-6	triglycerides
cell membranes	insulate	plant oils	twice
chylomicron	LDL cholesterol	rancidity	very low density
eicosanoids	lipase	satiety	lipoproteins (VLDL)
emulsifiers	liquid	saturated	water
energy	liver cells	Simplesse	whole milk
essential fatty acids	lymphatic system	small intestine	1 tablespoon
fat	no		

Check your answers using the summary for Chapter 6 in your textbook.

Answers to selected questions

IV. E. 1.
1. white rice - 0 grams of fat
2. green split pea soup - 5 grams
3. Triscuits - 9 grams
4. Snickers Bar - 12 grams
5. croissant - 13 grams
6. fried chicken - 14 grams
7. roast beef - 15 grams
8. eggs - 18 grams
9. peanuts - 20 grams
10. cheddar cheese - 21 grams (this is a major fat source in the American diet)

F.
1. high blood pressure, smoking, high serum cholesterol level
2. saturated fat*, cholesterol
3. eat less saturated fat; eat less cholesterol, eat less total fat, eat more soluble fiber

---

_B_   1.   Which group of foods is highest in fat?

    A. hamburger, french fries, and cupcake.
    B. margarine, salad dressing, and corn oil.
    C. cottage cheese, chicken, and soybeans.
    D. eggs, cheese, and milk.
    E. apple, spinach, and corn.

_C_   2.   If an 1800-kcalorie diet contains 100 grams of fat, the percentage of kcalories from the fat is:

    A. 20 %.   C. 50 %.
    B. 35 %.   D. 65 %.

_A_   3.   The three-carbon "backbone" found in all triglycerides is called:

    A. glycerol.   C. acetic acid.
    B. fatty acid.   D. stearic acid.

_C_   4.   Hydrogenation of fat does <u>NOT</u>:

    A. increase shelf life.
    B. make it harder.
    C. make it more unsaturated.
    D. reduce the tendency for oxidation.

_D_   5.   Moderate fish consumption is primarily related to a decreased risk for heart disease because it lowers:

    A. serum triglycerides.
    B. serum cholesterol.
    C. serum lipoproteins.
    D. blood clotting activity.

_B_   6.   If Jack Sprat truly could eat no fat, he would:

    A. eliminate his risk for cancer.
    B. not be able to make prostaglandins.
    C. necessarily have a low serum cholesterol level.
    D. have a high satiety value for his diet.

_A_   7.   Cholesterol:

    A. comes only from the animal food in our diet.
    B. must be eaten in the diet.
    C. is a breakdown product of lipids.
    D. when present in the diet, is the leading cause of strokes.

_C_   8.   The form of lipid in food is primarily in the form of:

    A. cholesterol.   C. triglycerides.
    B. fatty acids.   D. phospholipids.

_A_   9.   Which of the following is <u>NOT</u> an emulsifier?

    A. glycerol.   C. lecithin.
    B. bile acids.   D. diglycerides.

__A__   10.   Emulsifiers and micelles are related in that:

        A. an emulsifier forms a micelle.
        B. a micelle produces an emulsifier.
        C. both are classified as carbohydrates.
        D. both operate primarily in the stomach.

__A__   11.   Because lard is a solid at room temperature, most of its fatty acids are:

        A. long and saturated.
        B. short and saturated.
        C. long and unsaturated.
        D. short and unsaturated.

__C__   12.   A symptom of an essential fatty acid deficiency is:

        A. anemia.   C. skin rash.
        B. hair color changes.   D. loss of hearing.

__B__   13.   Bile acids are made from:

        A. glucose.   C. vitamin A.
        B. cholesterol.   D. prostaglandins.

__B__   14.   The three major risk factors for heart disease do <u>NOT</u> include:

        A. high serum cholesterol level.
        B. obesity.
        C. hypertension.
        D. smoking.

For questions 15 to 18, identify the following lipoproteins:

        A. chylomicron
        B. very low density lipoprotein
        C. low density lipoprotein
        D. high density lipoprotein

__A__   15.   main carrier of dietary triglyceride in the bloodstream
__C__   16.   highest in cholesterol content in terms of weight
__B__   17.   main carrier of triglyceride synthesized by the liver to body cells
__D__   18.   linked to decreased in heart disease risk

For questions 19 to 22, indicate a concentrated food source for the following (use each food only once):

__D__   19.   saturated fat   A. canola oil
__B__   20.   cholesterol   B. liver
__C__   21.   polyunsaturated fat   C. safflower oil
__A__   22.   monounsaturated fat   D. butter

Match the following terms:

__C__   23.   atherosclerosis   A. block in blood flow in brain
__B__   24.   myocardial infarction B. reduction in blood flow in the heart
__A__   25.   stroke   C. buildup of fatty material in arteries

__A__   26.   The lipid in the diet that most profoundly raises serum cholesterol levels is:

        A. saturated fat.   C. polyunsaturated fat.
        B. monounsaturated fat.   D. cholesterol.

Chapter 7
Proteins

I.   **Points to consider**

Chapter 7 is designed to allow you to:

1. Describe how amino acids make up proteins.

2. Distinguish between essential (indispensable) and nonessential (dispensable) amino acids.

3. Explain why adequate amounts of each of the essential amino acids are required for protein synthesis.

4. List six functions of protein in the body.

5. Calculate, when weight is given, the RDA for protein for an adult.

6. Describe what is represented by positive nitrogen balance, negative nitrogen balance, and nitrogen equilibrium.

7. Distinguish between high-quality and low-quality protein and the sources of each, as well as describe how two low-quality proteins can be complimentary for each other and in turn provide all the essential amino acids.

8. Describe how protein energy malnutrition can eventually lead to disease in the body.

II.   **Word parts**

Complete the following exercise using words in Chapter 7.

Word part	Meaning	Examples
amine	organic form of nitrogen	__________
a	without	__________
ost	bone	__________
ov	egg	__________

III.   **Flash cards**

Cut out and review the flash cards for this chapter in Appendix A.

IV.   Review and synthesis

A.   "The most nutrient-dense source of protein is water-packed tuna, which has over 80% of kcalories as protein." To review important concepts about protein digestion and absorption, imagine that for lunch you ate cheese pizza and drank a glass of 2% milk. Describe the digestion of the protein in the meal in each part of the digestive system. (197)

DIGESTIVE ACTIVITY

<u>Organ</u>

Mouth

Stomach

Small intestine

    Lumen (interior)

    Absorptive cells

____

The final end products of protein digestion are:

After absorption, at what organ does the major end product first arrive?

B.   1.   "Amino acids are the building blocks of proteins." The chemical elements (atoms) used to make amino acids are: (193)

a.   c.   e.

b.   d.

2.   "Amino acids are joined together in specific sequences to form distinct proteins. The sequential order of the amino acids determines a protein's configuration ." Outline in your own words what is meant by this statement. Define within this context the term "denature." (200)

C.   "Therefore, proteins truly do deserve their name, which means 'to come first.' Describe four roles proteins serve in the body. (201)

        a.

        b.

        c.

        d.

D.   1.   "Merely eating more protein does not guarantee a positive balance." Describe protein balance in practical terms. Then complete the following table. (204)

Positive protein balance is seen in:	Negative protein balance is seen in:

      2.   "Today the best estimate for the amount of protein required for nearly all adults is 0.8 grams of protein per kilogram of desirable body weight." Calculate your RDA for protein below. Desirable weight for heights are listed on the inside cover of your textbook. Recall that 2.2 pounds equals 1 kilogram. (205)

V.   Applying nutrition to your life

"In a healthy person the amount of dietary protein needed to maintain equilibrium can be determined by increasing protein intake, until intake just equals losses. This recommended amount works out to about 56 grams of protein a day for a 70-kilogram (154-pound) man and 44 grams of protein daily for a 55-kilogram (120-pound) woman." (205) Consult the list of foods you ate and recorded in Chapter 1 of the textbook. Use Appendix A in your textbook to calculate the number of grams of protein in each food item. Now, using the RDA for protein that you just calculated for yourself, did you meet your RDA for protein that day?

<u>Foods</u>   <u>Grams of protein</u>

Breakfast

Lunch

Dinner

Total grams of protein ________________________

VI.   Chapter 7 summary

Fill in the blanks using the words listed at the end of this summary.

__________ are the building blocks of proteins. Amino acids contain a very usable form of

__________ for us. Of the 20 major types of amino acids found in food, 9 are __________ to consume and

11 can be synthesized by the body.

High quality, also called "__________," protein foods contain ample amounts of all 9 essential

amino acids. Animal foods typically supply all of them in close to the right amounts. __________, also

called "incomplete" protein, lack sufficient amino acids. This is typical of __________ foods, especially cereal

grains.

Supplementing the diet with large amounts of individual amino acids can lead to a __________ of

harmful levels.

Protein digestion begins primarily in the __________, producing breakdown products called

__________. In the small intestine peptones separate into small __________ and amino acids. These are absorbed into the absorptive cells of the __________ and travel via the __________ to the __________.

Individual amino acids are __________ together to form proteins. The sequential order of amino acids determines the protein's ultimate form, and in turn __________. If the three-dimensional shape of the protein eventually formed is unfolded or __________ by treatment with heat, acid or alkaline solutions, or other processes, the protein loses its biological activity. Essential body components, such as muscles, __________, transport proteins, visual pigments, __________, some hormones, and immune bodies are made up of proteins. The RDA for protein for adults is __________ grams per kilogram of desirable body weight. The typical American man consumes about __________ grams of protein daily and __________ consume closer to 70 grams daily. Thus, the American diet generally supplies plenty of __________.

Animal meats are the most nutrient-dense sources of protein. __________ contains 85% of its kcalories as protein, plant foods generally contain less than __________ of their kcalories as proteins; however, __________ provide much protein when regularly part of a diet and contribute to a high quality protein for a meal if eaten with grain products. These sources are critical for __________ diets.

Undernutrition occasionally leads to __________ and marasmus. Kwashiorkor results primarily from a poor __________ and protein intake, in combination with concurrent disease and infection. __________ results primarily from basic __________ -- a negligible intake of both protein and kcalories is seen.

Use the following words to complete the summary

amino acids	kwashiorkor	portal vein
build up	legumes	protein
complete	linked	starvation
connective tissue	liver	stomach
denatured	low quality	vegetarian
enzymes	marasmus	villi
essential	nitrogen	water-packed tuna
function	peptides	women
kcalorie	peptones	0.8
	plant	20%
		90

Check your answers using the Summary for Chapter 7 in your textbook.

Cover the answers on your initial attempt.

__B__ 1. A buffer helps:

A. emulsify fats.
B. maintain a constant pH in a solution.
C. speed chemical reactions.
D. protect against plaque build-up in the arteries.

__D__ 2. Which of the following is definitely not a protein?

A. antibody.   C. tendon.
B. enzyme.   D. glycogen.

__A__ 3. Peptide bonds are formed:

A. by excluding water molecules.
B. by excluding hydrogen atoms.
C. by making esters.
D. when developing secondary structure.

__B__ 4. Nonessential amino acids:

A. are not needed by the body.
B. are not needed in the diet.
C. are not needed daily, but weekly.
D. are found in only incomplete proteins.

__B__ 5. The denaturing of protein:

A. destroys its amino acid order.
B. happens in the stomach.
C. increases its enzyme activity.
D. forms an emulsifier.

__B__ 6. The order of amino acids in a specific protein determines its:

A. kcalorie content.
B. function in the body.
C. biological value.
D. ability to form glucose.

__D__ 7. Vegetarians who eat no animal products or nutrient-fortified products should supplement their diets with:

A. vitamin C.   C. vitamin A.
B. magnesium.   D. vitamin B-12.

__B__ 8. Incomplete proteins:

A. do not follow the "all-or-none law."
B. are characteristic of plant foods.
C. are characteristic of animal foods.
D. are characteristic of snack foods.

__C__ 9. The RDA for protein of a 60-kilogram (132-pound) woman is:

A. 36 grams.   D. 54 grams.
B. 42 grams.   E. 60 grams.
C. 48 grams.

_D_ 10. Which is <u>NOT</u> true about kwashiorkor?

A. Protein needs are generally not met.
B. The child appears plump due to edema.
C. The child is at a high risk for infections.
D. The affected person is usually a very young infant.

_A_ 11. In marasmus:

A. the child is often bottle-fed from birth.
B. protein needs are met.
C. muscle wasting is present, but it is hidden by edema.
D. preschool children, not infants, are typically affected.

_A_ 12. Which of the following is <u>NOT</u> a protein?

A. maltose.   C. insulin.
B. hemoglobin.   D. collagen.

_B_ 13. Which of the following does <u>NOT</u> provide mixtures of amino acids that are well balanced for humans?

A. corn and refried beans.
B. jello.
C. eggs.
D. macaroni and cheese.

_B_ 14. A good protein intake recommendation is ______ of total kcalories:

A. 5% to 10%.   C. 15% to 20%.
B. 10% to 15%.   D. 20% to 25%.

_B_ 15. Clinical edema occurs when:

A. the plasma protein level is increased.
B. the plasma protein level is decreased.
C. the red cell number decreases.
D. there is no change in plasma hemoglobin.

_D_ 16. The exchange group that contributes no protein is:

A. milk.   C. vegetable.
B. starch/bread.   D. fruit.

_B_ 17. The chemical element (atom) found in all proteins, but not usually in fats or carbohydrates, is:

A. carbon.   C. hydrogen.
B. nitrogen.   D. oxygen.

_D_ 18. An essential (indispensable) amino acid:

A. forms a complete protein.
B. is needed only by growing infants and children.
C. may prevent dermatitis.
D. cannot by synthesized by the body in sufficient amounts to meet the
   body's needs.

_C_ 19. During pregnancy, nitrogen balance should be:

A. negative.   B. in equilibrium.   C. positive.

| D | 20. | If a person takes in more protein than the body needs, the excess protein will be: |

A. excreted in the urine.
B. converted to fat energy and stored in adipocytes.
C. used to provide energy for the body if needed.
D. B and C.

| C | 21. | The RDA for protein is increased: |

A. during mental stress.
B. after age 50.
C. during pregnancy and lactation.
D. whenever physical activity is increased.

| A | 22. | One would expect to see a negative protein balance: |

A. when certain hormones, such as thyroid hormone and cortisol, are released in excess amounts.
B. during pregnancy.
C. as one recovers from an illness.
D. in any healthy human being.

| B | 23. | Proteins supply 2 to 5% of the energy the body uses, but is not the primary source cells use because: |

A. the decreased amount of energy per gram available compared to carbohydrates.
B. the amount of metabolism and processing required by the liver and kidneys.
C. the inability of the body to make glucose from amino acids.
D. the complex planning required to obtain all nine essential amino acids in a typical diet.

| C | 24. | Urea is synthesized from amino (NH) groups mostly in which tissue? |

A. blood   C. liver
B. kidneys   D. small intestine

| C | 25. | Approximately 32% to 43% of dietary protein must supply essential amino acids for: |

A. the very elderly.
B. pregnant women.
C. infants.
D. athletes.
E. vegetarians.

Chapter 8
Vitamins

I.   **Points to consider**

Chapter 8 is designed to allow you to:

1.   Define the term vitamin.

2.   Classify the vitamins according to whether they are fat-soluble or water-soluble.

3.   List the major functions and deficiency symptoms for each fat-soluble vitamin.

4.   List the major functions and deficiency symptoms for each water-soluble vitamin.

5.   List three important food sources for each fat-soluble vitamin.

6.   List three important food sources for each water-soluble vitamin.

7.   Describe toxicity symptoms from excess consumption of fat-soluble vitamins and certain water-soluble vitamins.

8.   Distinguish between vitamins and nonvitamins, such as choline and taurine.

9.   Evaluate the pros and cons of use of vitamin and mineral supplements.

10.   Describe some cancer-causing mechanisms and describe how diet and nutrition are related to their minimization.

II.   **Word parts**

Complete the following exercise using words in Chapter 8.

Word Part	Meaning	Example
xero	dry	_____________
osteo	bone	_____________
mal	poor	_____________
oid	like, resemble	_____________
malacia	softened	_____________
blast	immature cell	_____________
osis	condition of	_____________
cyte	cell	_____________

III.   Flash cards

Cut out and review the flash cards for this chapter in Appendix A.

IV.   Review and synthesis

A.   "Vitamins can be defined as carbon-containing substances that the body must obtain, in only small amounts, to maintain health." Differentiate between the classes of vitamins using the terms in parentheses. Use one term twice if appropriate. (225; 242)

	<u>Fat-soluble</u>	<u>Water-soluble</u>
Absorbed into (blood or lymph)		
Excess (easily excreted or poorly excreted)		
Excesses (often toxic or not often toxic)		
Generally (form or do not form) coenzymes		
Generally (stable or unstable) during cooking		

B.   "The water-soluble vitamins, particularly thiamin, vitamin C, and folate, can be destroyed with improper storage and excessive cooking." Provide suggestions for retaining the maximum amount of vitamins when storing, preparing, and cooking vegetables. (242)

    1.   Storing vegetables

        a.

        b.

    2.   Preparing and cooking vegetables

        a.

        b.

        c.

        d.

C.	"For vitamin A, the preferred unit of measurement is the retinol equivalent (RE)." (230)

1.	The provitamin forms of vitamin A are found in ___________________ foods, whereas

	the already active forms of vitamin A are found in ______________ foods.

2.	The RDAs (from inside cover of textbook) for men and women ages 19 to 50 years for vitamin A are:

	men ________________RE		women ________________RE

D.	"The net result of vitamin D hormone action is to increase calcium and phosphorus deposition in bones." Describe how rickets could develop in childhood. (232)

E.	"Vitamin E, a fat-soluble antioxidant, mostly resides in cell membranes." (235)

1.	How does vitamin E protect fats from breakdown?

2.	What would be one health consequence if vitamin E was lacking in one's diet?

3.	How does the mineral selenium spare some of the body's need for vitamin E?

F.   "The amount of vitamin K in our diets alone is generally about five times higher than our needs." (238)

1.   List two groups of people who may develop vitamin K deficiency. Briefly explain your reasons for listing these groups.

a.

b.

2.   Describe the most likely result from a vitamin K deficiency. Why would these symptoms appear?

G.   "This shows how limited the body's stores of thiamin are and how important it is to consume thiamin-rich foods daily." Discuss two reasons, besides poor body storage of thiamin, why a two week alcohol binge could lead to a thiamin deficiency. (241)

H.   "It is quite easy to take a toxic dose." Dispel the notion that high doses of all water-soluble vitamins are safe. (246)

I.   "Probably the most important role of the folate coenzymes is helping to form DNA." What tissues are first affected by a folate deficiency? Why? (247)

J.   "Vitamins yield no energy for the body." To review the fat-soluble vitamins and water-soluble vitamins, complete the following chart. (Use Tables 8-2 and 8-3 in your textbook to check your answers).

	Major function(s)	Likely result of a long-term deficiency	Nutrient-dense food sources	Likelihood for toxicity and possible result(s)
Vitamin A				
Vitamin D				
Vitamin E				
Vitamin K				
Thiamin				
Niacin				
Riboflavin				
Pantothenic acid				
Biotin				
Vitamin B-6				
Folate				
Vitamin B-12				
Vitamin C				

V.   **Applying nutrition to your life**

Do you really need a vitamin supplement?

Read the nutrition labels of five food items you eat tomorrow. If you eat breakfast cereal, make sure you include that food in your calculations. Also, include foods you feel are especially nutritious parts of your diet. Write down the percentage of the U.S. RDA for the following water-soluble vitamins. Now total the amounts for each vitamin.

Foods	1	2	3	4	5	Total
Thiamin						_________
Niacin						_________
Riboflavin						_________
Vitamin B-6						_________
Folate						_________
Vitamin B-12						_________
Vitamin C						_________

Did you meet your needs as predicted by the U.S. RDA (100%) that day for all the vitamins listed?

Note: If there are large gaps between your intake and 100%, review the diet analysis you did for Chapter 2 in your textbook before deciding if a vitamin supplement is needed. Typically this exercise alone will convince you one is not needed.

VI.   **Chapter 8 summary**

Fill in the blanks using the words listed at the end of this summary.

______________ are compounds we need daily in small amounts from foods. They yield no

___________ themselves, but many contribute to energy-yielding chemical reactions in the body and

promote growth and development. Many vitamins act as ____________, helping enzymes function.

Vitamins A, D, E, and K are fat-soluble, whereas the B vitamins and vitamin C are ____________.

Fat-soluble vitamins are absorbed along with dietary fat and are more poorly excreted from the body than water-soluble vitamins.

Vitamin A consists of a family of compounds that includes several forms of ___________ vitamin A. ___________, such as beta-carotene, function as antioxidants and can also yield vitamin A. Vitamin A helps maintain mucus-forming cells, _________, proper immune function, and normal growth. Vitamin A is found in liver and fish oils; carotenes are especially plentiful in dark green and orange vegetables. Vitamin A can be quite ___________, even when taken at just 5 to 10 times the RDA.

Vitamin D is both a ___________ and a vitamin. Human skin synthesizes it using sunshine and a cholesterol-like substance. If we don't spend enough time in the sun, foods such as fish oils and fortified ___________ must supply the vitamin. The active hormone form of vitamin D helps regulate blood calcium levels by influencing calcium absorption from the ___________. It also helps to regulate bone metabolism. Children who don't get enough vitamin D may develop ___________, and adults with inadequate amounts in the body develop _______________. Vitamin D is a very toxic substance. An intake just 2.5 to ___________ times the RDA can cause problems.

Vitamin E functions primarily as an ___________. By donating electrons to electron-seeking (oxidizing) compounds, it neutralizes them. This shields cell membranes and red blood cells from ___________. Vitamin E is plentiful in ___________.

___________ helps blood clot. About half the vitamin K absorbed each day comes from ___________ synthesis in the intestine, and the other half comes from foods, primarily ___________ vegetables. Vitamin K is poorly stored in the body, but our dietary intake alone is usually ___________.

Thiamin, ___________, and niacin play key roles as coenzymes in energy-yielding reactions. They help ___________ carbohydrates, fats, and proteins. ___________ and a poor diet can create deficiencies of these three nutrients. ___________ products are common sources of all three of these vitamins.

Pantothenic acid, which participates in many aspects of cell metabolism, is widely distributed among foods. Biotin, which participates in ___________ production, fat synthesis, and DNA synthesis, can be synthesized by bacteria in the intestine. We probably synthesize about ___________ our

requirement for biotin. The rest comes from foods such as eggs and ___________.

Vitamin B-6 performs a vital role in protein metabolism, especially in synthesizing nonessential

___________. It also helps synthesize ___________ and performs other metabolic roles. Headaches,

anemia, ___________, and vomiting result from a B-6 deficiency. Regular consumption of

___________ protein foods, cauliflower, and broccoli provides needed vitamin B-6. Taking high doses

-- greater than 12 times the RDA -- causes malfunction of the ___________ system.

Folate plays an important role in _________ synthesis. Symptoms of a deficiency are generally

poor cell division in various areas of the body, anemia, ___________ inflammation, diarrhea, and poor

growth. Excellent food sources are leafy vegetables, organ meats, and _________ juice. Since great

amounts of folate can be lost in cooking, a healthy diet should emphasize ___________ or lightly

cooked vegetables.

Vitamin B-12 is needed to metabolize folate and to maintain the ___________ surrounding

nerves. A deficiency results in _________ (because of its relationship to folate) and nerve degeneration.

___________ people often absorb vitamin B-12 inefficiently. If so, they benefit from monthly injections

of the vitamin. For others, a ___________ is unlikely because vitamin B-12 is highly concentrated in

animal foods. Vitamin B-12 does not occur naturally in ___________ foods. ___________ need a

supplemental source.

___________ is used mainly to synthesize collagen, a major protein for building connective

tissue. A vitamin C deficiency results in ___________, which is evidenced by poor wound healing,

pinpoint hemorrhages in the skin, and bleeding gums. Vitamin C also enhances ___________

absorption. Fresh fruits and vegetables, especially ___________ fruits, are generally good sources.

Nutrition scientists generally agree that most people can obtain needed vitamins and minerals

from a varied, _________ diet. If you still think you need _________, talk to a registered dietitian

and/or your physician first because there is some risk from consuming even typical forms.

____________ is the second leading cause of death for adults in the United States; it affects different types of ____________ and arises from many different causes. The process begins with an alteration in DNA, the ____________ material in our cells. There are many ways to alter DNA, such as radiation from the sun, both natural and man-made chemicals, and the insertion of viral genes into human cells. Both ____________ and physical inactivity are linked to increased risk for many types of cancer.

Use the following words to complete the summary

alcoholism	enriched grain	plant oils
amino acids	fresh	preformed
anemia	genetic	riboflavin
animal	glucose	rickets
antioxidant	green, leafy	scurvy
bacterial	half	sufficient
balanced	hormone	tongue
breakdown	insulation	toxic
cells	intestine	vegans
cancer	iron	vision
carotenes	metabolize	vitamin and
cheese	milk	mineral
citrus	nausea	supplements
coenzymes	nervous	vitamins
deficiency	neurotransmitters	vitamin C
DNA	obesity	vitamin K
elderly	orange	water-soluble
energy	osteomalacia	5
	plant	

Check your answers using the summary for Chapter 8 in your textbook and the next page of this <u>Study Guide</u> for the last six answers.

VII.   Practice examination

Cover the answers on your initial attempt.

<u>C</u>   1.   The first symptom(s) of scurvy are:

A. dental caries.
B. depression and anxiety.
C. pinpoint hemorrhages under the skin.
D. pernicious anemia.

<u>B</u>   2.   Vitamin C is essential in the synthesis of a hydroxyproline residue found in:

A. ascorbic acid.   C. leukocytes.
B. collagen.   D. hemoglobin.

<u>B</u>   3.   Which of these meals lacks vitamin C?

A. corned beef, cabbage, fried potatoes, and milk
B. roast beef, carrots, noodles, and tea
C. spaghetti with tomato sauce, meatball, garlic bread, and diet soda
D. roast beef, broccoli, noodles, and coffee

<u>D</u>   4.   A deficiency of either of these two vitamins produces a similar type of anemia:

A. riboflavin and niacin.
B. thiamin and riboflavin.
C. pantothenic acid and biotin.
D. vitamin B-12 and folate.

<u>C</u>   5.   Choline is:

A. an enzyme.   C. part of lecithin.
B. part of bile.   D. a vitamin.

<u>C</u>   6.   Folate is found in small amounts in many foods, but the best sources are:

A. whole grain cereals.
B. cheese, eggs, and cream.
C. leafy green vegetables and some fruits.
D. raw sugar, honey, and molasses.

__C__   7.   The two foods high in vitamin B-6 are:

A. whole grains and vegetable oils.
B. citrus fruits and vegetable oils.
C. meat and dairy products.
D. orange fruits and vegetables.

__B__   8.   Vitamin B-6 participates in:

A. iron absorption.
B. amino acid and protein metabolism.
C. release of energy from minerals.
D. utilization of calcium and phosphorus.

__D__   9.   Alcohol interferes greatly with __________ absorption.

A. pantothenic acid
B. riboflavin
C. niacin
D. thiamin

__D__   10.   The major sources of riboflavin in the American diet are:

A. whole grains.
B. green leafy vegetables.
C. citrus fruits and tomatoes.
D. dairy products.

__C__   11.   A high intake of folate is dangerous because it:

A. means the person is eating too much protein.
B. is easily stored in the body.
C. can "mask" pernicious anemia.
D. increases vitamin B-12 needs.

__C__   12.   Thiamin is used for:

A. formation of polysaccharides.
B. formation of red blood cells.
C. energy release from nutrients.
D. collagen formation.

__A__   13.   Each of the B vitamins functions as a(n):

A. part of a coenzyme.
B. electrolyte.
C. anticoagulant.
D. source of energy.

__C__   14.   Pernicious anemia is primarily caused by a defect in:

A. vitamin B-12 intake.
B. vitamin B-12 excretion.
C. vitamin B-12 absorption.
D. vitamin B-12 interconversion.

__A__   15.   __________ may be lacking in the diet of strict vegetarians (vegans).

A. Vitamin B-12
B. Thiamin
C. Riboflavin
D. Niacin

_D_ 16.   Pantothenic acid is a part of the structure of:

A. pyruvate.   C. glycogen.
B. cobalamin.   D. coenzyme A.

_D_ 17.   Vitamins may be defined as:

A. inorganic compounds in food needed in small amounts for growth and
   maintenance of health.
B. organic compounds formed by the endocrine glands and necessary for growth
   and maintenance of health.
C. catalysts for hormones.
D. organic compounds in food needed in small amounts for growth and
   maintenance of health.

_C_ 18.   The only foods that generally provide ample amounts of vitamin C are:

A. meats.   C. vegetables and fruits.
B. milk and cheese.   D. breads and cereals.

_B_ 19.   Biotin is used for:

A. glucose absorption.   C. fatty acid metabolism.
B. urea production.   D. emulsification.

_A_ 20.   Which of the following statements is true for niacin?

A. It can be synthesized in the body from tryptophan.
B. It is an antioxidant.
C. It is water-soluble and therefore safe to administer in large doses.
D. It can be used to successfully cure anemia.

Match the vitamin to the appropriate deficiency disease.

_C_	21.	scurvy	A. riboflavin
_D_	22.	beriberi	B. niacin
_F_	23.	megaloblastic anemia	C. vitamin C
_E_	24.	pernicious anemia	D. thiamin
_B_	25.	pellagra	E. vitamin B-12
_A_	26.	cheilosis	F. folate
_H_	27.	vitamin A	G. red blood cell hemolysis
_I_	28.	vitamin D	H. xerophthalmia
_G_	29.	vitamin E	I. osteomalacia

__B__   30.   Vitamin K is needed in the body for:

       A. enzyme action.   C. energy production.
       B. blood clotting.   D. strengthening bones and teeth.

__D__   31.   Identify one function of vitamin D:

       A. necessary for glucose metabolism.
       B. prevents scurvy.
       C. acts as an antioxidant.
       D. aids in the absorption of calcium.

__D__   32.   Which of the following substitutes for some of our need for vitamin E?

       A. sodium   C. silver
       B. sulfur   D. selenium

__C__   33.   One of the last signs of vitamin A deficiency is:

       A. anemia.   C. blindness.
       B. osteoporosis.   D. hemorrhage.

__D__   34.   The vitamin synthesized by bacteria in the intestine is:

       A. E.   B. D.   C. A.   D. K.

__A__   35.   Which of the following is <u>not</u> generally a true statement about fat-soluble vitamins?

       A. Excess amounts are easily excreted from the body.
       B. They can be consumed less frequently than the water-soluble vitamins.
       C. They are bound to proteins when traveling in the blood.
       D. They may accumulate to toxic levels in the body.

__D__   36.   Identify the best sources of beta-carotene:

       A. whole grains, nuts, seeds, egg yolk, and plant oils.
       B. lean meat, poultry, fish, and legumes.
       C. corn, peas, beans, peaches, and asparagus.
       D. pumpkin, carrots, squash, sweet potatoes, and apricots.

__C__   37.   Which of the following symptoms would indicate a vitamin D deficiency in infants and young children?

       A. abnormally high blood calcium levels
       B. rupture of red blood cells
       C. bowed legs
       D. abnormally low blood calcium levels

__D__   38.   Which of the following is <u>not</u> a good source of vitamin D?

       A. sunshine   C. fortified milk and margarine
       B. fatty fish   D. fruit, vegetables, and whole grains

_D_   39.   Vitamin K is found in:

A. seafood, iodized salt, and dairy products.
B. citrus fruits, cantaloupe, seeds, and nuts.
C. whole-grain cereals, milk, and cheese.
D. green leafy vegetables and broccoli.

_B_   40.   Vitamin E functions in the body:

A. for maintenance of vision and health of skin, as well as growth of nails and bones.
B. as an antioxidant to prevent cell damage.
C. to calcify bones and teeth.
D. to supply energy and spare protein.

_C_   41.   The Council of Scientific Affairs of the American Medical Association recommends taking no more than _______ to _______ of the adult U.S. RDA for vitamins.

A. 100% to 150%   C. 50% to 150%
B. 60% to 120%   D. 25% to 50%

_B_   42.   All adults should faithfully take a multivitamin at least once a day in order to prevent illness of becoming deficient in many nutrients.

A. True   B. False

Chapter 9
Water and Minerals

I.   **Points to consider**

Chapter 9 is designed to allow you to:

1. Classify the minerals as major or trace minerals.

2. List conditions of the body, dietary factors, and other pertinent relationships that influence the absorption, retention, and availability of specific minerals.

3. List and briefly explain the functions of water in the body.

4. List key functions of the major and trace minerals.

5. Identify possible deficiency and toxicity symptoms associated with the major and trace minerals.

6. List three food sources for each of the major and trace minerals.

7. Describe the processes involving minerals that aid in maintaining bone health as well as those that aid in control of blood pressure.

8. Evaluate the use of mineral supplements with respect to their benefits and hazards to the body.

II.   **Word parts**

Complete the following exercise using words in Chapter 9.

Word part	Meaning	Examples
penia	deficiency	_______________
intra	inside	_______________
extra	outside	_______________
tens	to stretch	_______________
myo	muscle	_______________
hem	blood	_______________
emia	in blood	_______________
chrom	color	_______________
goit	throat	_______________

III.   **Flash cards**

Cut out and review the flash cards for this chapter in Appendix A.

IV.   **Review and synthesis**

A.   "Minerals, like water, are vital to health." Explain how balance and variety in the diet, and body promote optimum mineral absorption. (273)

B.   "Depending on how much fat has been stored, an adult can survive for about 8 weeks without eating food but only a few days without drinking water." There are several sources of water, several routes of excretion, and many functions of water in the body. Sort the items in the box into the correct categories. (266)

Sources	Functions	Excretion
_______	_______	_______
_______	_______	_______
_______	_______	_______
	_______	_______

1. evaporation
2. feces
3. solid food
4. beverages
5. acid-base balance
6. solvent
7. perspiration
8. temperature regulation
9. medium for transport
10. urine
11. metabolic water

C. "If we ate only unprocessed foods and added no salt, sodium intake would be about 500 milligrams per day." (275)

  1. Compare the sodium contents (per 100 kcalories) of foods in the Food Guide Pyramid using Appendix A in your textbook.

<u>Sodium (Na)</u>
(mg per 100 kcalories)

   __________ Milk (whole)
   __________ Cheese (cheddar)
           Vegetable
   __________ leafy (spinach)
   __________ other (corn)
   __________ Fruit (apple)
   __________ Breads and Cereals (enriched bread)
   __________ Meat (steak)
   __________ Egg
   __________ Fat (use margarine)

Note: 500 milligrams is the minimum requirement for health.

  2. To what extent does sodium enter in the diet from natural foods versus manufactured foods, based on these values?

D. "Because the bones are not as dense as normal bones, osteoporosis can lead to a decrease in height, hip fractures in old age, and eventual loss of teeth." (280)

  1. List 3 factors associated with bone maintenance versus bone loss.

<u>Maintenance</u>	<u>Loss</u>
a.	a.
b.	b.
c.	c.

2.	Based on this information, what recommendations might you make to a 10-year-old girl to decrease her risk for osteoporosis in later years? (285)

E.	"Minerals are vital to the functioning of many body processes." (288) List two major minerals that:

1.	help maintain bone mass in the body.

a.

b.

2.	help maintain water balance in the body.

a.

b.

3.	help promote nerve function in the body.

a.

b.

4.	are necessary for the contraction and relaxation of the muscles.

a.

b.

See page 112 of this <u>Study Guide</u> for possible answers.

5.   Place a check mark when a food group makes an important contribution for a major
        mineral. Refer to Table 9-4 if you need help.

Food Group	Na	K	Cl	Ca	P	Mg
Milk and cheese						
Meat, fish, poultry, and beans						
Fruits and vegetables						
Breads and cereals						

F.   1.   "While minerals may be present in foods, they are not 'bioavailable' unless a body can
            absorb them. The ability to absorb minerals from a diet depends on many factors." List
            4 factors that increase and 4 factors that decrease iron absorption. (289)

Increase   Decrease

a.   a.

b.   b.

c.   c.

d.   d.

2.   "More people have an iron deficiency than iron-deficiency anemia, especially in
        America." Compare the effects of iron deficiency on the body to those resulting from
        iron-deficiency anemia. (290)

3.   Provide four suggestions for increasing a poor iron intake. (291)

    a.   c.

    b.   d.

G.   "Men drafted from the Pacific Northwest and the Great Lakes Region of the United States had a much higher rate of goiter than men from other areas of the country. The soils in these areas have very low iodide contents." (295)

    1.   One of the symptoms of iodide deficiency is an enlargement of the thyroid gland. Why does this gland enlarge as a result of this deficiency?

    2.   Briefly discuss the main reason why iodide deficiency is now rare in the United States.

H. "Information about trace minerals is perhaps the most rapidly expanding area of knowledge in nutrition." Complete the following table. (299)

Trace mineral	Major function(s)	Likely result of long-term deficiency	Good food sources	Likelihood for toxicity and possible results
Zinc				
Copper				
Selenium				
Fluoride				

V. **Applying nutrition to your life**

"We consume about 1 liter (1 quart) per day of water a day in various liquids. Foods supply another liter of fluid; many fruits, vegetables, and beverages are more than 80% water. Water as a by-product of metabolism provides approximately 350 milliliters (1-1/2 cups of additional water). (269) Use your diet record from in the textbook to examine your beverage intake in terms of amount and kcalories supplied (1 cup = 8 fluid ounces).

<u>Beverage</u>	<u>Amount (cups) for the day</u>	<u>kcalories</u>
Water		----------
Milk		
Fruit juices		

Soft drinks
  regular
  diet		

Coffee/tea		
Hot chocolate		
Sports drinks		
Alcoholic beverages		
TOTAL	____________ total cups	____________ total kcalories
	____________ total milliliters (cups x 240)	

---

1.   What was your primary beverage?

2.   Were the energy-containing beverages generally nutritious beverages or non-nutritious beverages?

3.   Did you meet the general guidelines of 1 milliliter of fluid per total kcalories expended for the day? What one change do you think is needed in your beverage habits?

Fill in the blanks using the words listed at the end of this summary.

Water constitutes ________ of the human body. Its unique chemical properties enable it to dissolve substances, as well as serve as a medium for chemical reactions, thermoregulation, and __________. For adults, daily water needs are estimated at 1 milliliter per kcalorie _______. Many _______ are vital for sustaining life. For humans, animal products are the most bioavailable source of minerals. Supplements of minerals exceeding 150% of the U.S. RDA should be taken only under a physician's supervision, since _______ and nutrient interactions are a likely possibility.

Sodium, the major positive ion of the _______ fluid, is vital in fluid balance and nerve impulse transmission. The American diet provides abundant ________ through processed foods and table salt. About 10% to 15% of the adult population is ________ and is at risk for developing hypertension from consuming excessive sodium.

Potassium, the major positive ion of the ________ fluid, functions similarly to sodium. Milk, _________, and vegetables are good sources. ________ is the major negative ion in extracellular fluid. It is important in digestion as part of gastric _________ and in immune function. Table salt supplies most of the chloride in our diets.

Calcium forms a vital part of bone structure and is also very important in ________, muscle contraction, nerve transmission, and cell control. Calcium absorption is enhanced by stomach acid and the active ________ hormone. Dairy products are important calcium sources. Bone loss in _________ is linked to low calcium intake. Women are particularly at risk for this condition and should get plenty of calcium and _______ regularly. ________ replacement at menopause is currently the most accepted way to stop significant adult bone loss in women after menopause.

________ aids enzyme function and forms part of energy-containing molecules, cell membranes, and bone. It is efficiently absorbed, and deficiencies are rare, although there is concern about the intake by _______ women. Good food sources are dairy products, bakery products, and meats. Sulfur is incorporated into certain vitamins and _________. Magnesium is a mineral found mostly in plants. It is important for _________ and heart function and as an activator for many enzymes. Whole grains (bran portion), vegetables, _______, seeds, milk, and meats are good food sources.

Iron absorption depends mainly on the form of iron present and the body's need for it. _________ iron from animal sources is better absorbed than the nonheme iron obtained primarily from plant sources. Consuming _________ simultaneously with iron will increase nonheme absorption. Iron operates mainly in synthesizing _________ and myoglobin and in the action of the immune system. Women are at greater risk for developing iron deficiency, which decreases blood hemoglobin level and red blood cell number. When this condition in severe enough to decrease the amount of oxygen carried in the blood, iron-deficiency _________ develops. Iron toxicity usually results from a genetic disorder called _________.

Zinc aids in the action of over 200 enzymes that are important for growth, development, immune function, _________, and taste. A zinc deficiency results in poor growth, loss of appetite, reduced sense of taste and smell, _______ loss, and a persistent rash. Zinc is best absorbed from animal sources. The most nutrient-dense sources of zinc are oysters, _______, crab, and beef. Good plant sources are whole grains, peanuts, and beans. Copper is important for _______metabolism, collagen cross-bonding, and other functions. A _______ deficiency can result in an iron deficiency type of anemia. Copper is found mainly in some sea foods, legumes, and _________.

An important role of selenium is in decreasing action of _________ compounds. In this way, selenium acts along with vitamin E. Muscle pain, _________, and heart disease may result from a selenium deficiency. Meats, especially _______ meats, eggs, fish, and shellfish are good animal sources of selenium. Good plant sources include grains and seeds. Iodide forms part of the _______ hormones. A lack of dietary iodide results in the development of an enlarged thyroid gland or _________. Iodized salt is a good food source. Fluoride incorporated into teeth during development makes them resistant to _________. Most Americans receive the bulk of their fluoride from fluoridated _________ and toothpaste.

Chromium helps regulate _________ uptake by cells. Egg yolks and whole grains are good sources of chromium. Manganese and ___________ are used by various enzymes. Human needs for other trace minerals are so low that deficiencies are uncommon.

Blood pressure is expressed by two numbers. The higher number represents ___________ blood pressure, the pressure in the arteries when the heart actively pumps blood. The second value is for ___________ pressure, the arterial pressure when the heart is relaxed. ____________ is defined as sustained high blood pressure, usually with systolic pressure exceeding __________ mm Hg or diastolic blood pressure exceeding 90 mm Hg. A variety of factors affecting blood pressure include age, atherosclerosis, ___________, race, and sodium intake.

Use the following words to complete the summary

amino acids	extracellular	lubrication	sodium-sensitive
anemia	fruits	minerals	systolic
blood clotting	glucose	molybdenum	thyroid
chloride	goiter	muscle wasting	toxicity
copper	hair	nerve	vitamin C
dental caries	heme	nuts	vitamin D
diastolic	hemochromatosis	obesity	water
elderly	hemoglobin	organ	whole grains
electron-seeking	hypertension	osteoporosis	wound healing
estrogen	hydrochloric acid	phosphorus	50% to 70%
exercise	intracellular	shrimp	140
expended	iron	sodium	

Check your answers using the summary for Chapter 9 in your textbook, and the next page of this <u>Study Guide</u> for the last seven answers.

VII. Practice examination

Cover the answers on your initial attempt.

Match the letter to the appropriate mineral.

H	1.	cobalt	A.	aids transport of oxygen
B	2.	copper	B.	aids in iron metabolism
D	3.	chromium	C.	associated with control of metabolic rate
C	4.	iodide	D.	contributes to normal metabolism of blood glucose
A	5.	iron	E.	needed for wound healing
F	6.	manganese	F.	needed for activity of enzymes used in
G	7.	selenium		carbohydrate metabolism
E	8.	zinc	G.	works with vitamin E
I	9.	fluoride	H.	part of vitamin B-12
			I.	strengthens tooth crystal

D 10. Iron is rapidly depleted from the body during:

A. vigorous exercise.
B. high calcium absorption.
C. rapid weight loss.
D. blood loss.

A 11. The most reliable food sources of zinc is (are):

A. meats and seafood.
B. orange juice.
C. dark green vegetables.
D. iodized salt.

B 12. Iron absorption from plant sources can be increased by _______ in the meal.

A. phytic acid   C. phosphates
B. vitamin C   D. fiber

A 13. Which of the following does not have antioxidant properties?

A. zinc   C. vitamin E
B. vitamin C   D. selenium

A 14. If an adult male is anemic, the first cause physicians suspect is:

A. a bleeding ulcer.   C. a poor diet.
B. cirrhosis of the liver. D. kidney disease.

_D_   15.   Iodide deficiency results in:

A. anemia.   C. osteomalacia.
B. scurvy.   D. goiter.

_B_   16.   High intakes of iron in certain people can lead to:

A. anemia.   C. hypertension.
B. liver damage.   D. ulcers.

_D_   17.   Calcium is used in the body for:

A. enzyme regulation in cells.
B. excitability of nerves and muscles.
C. blood coagulation.
D. all of the above.

_B_   18.   About how much water does the average adult take in as fluid and then excrete as urine per day?

A. 1 cup   B. 4 cups   C. 10 cups   D. 20 cups

_A_   19.   Calcium absorption is aided by:

A. vitamin D.
B. phosphorus and fiber.
C. oxalate and phytate.
D. all of the above.

_A_   20.   The mineral that is part of the green pigment, chlorophyll, is:

A. magnesium.   B. calcium.   C. iron.   D. selenium.

_B_   21.   If enough calcium is not consumed:

A. heart rate will slow.
B. calcium will be removed from bone.
C. nerve impulses will cease.
D. caries will occur in the teeth.

_A_   22.   Which of the following is not a function of water in the body?

A. acts as an antioxidant
B. allows for the excretion of wastes
C. allows us to transport many nutrients
D. helps dissolve certain substances

_D_   23.   The sodium content of the diet of most Americans is _______ the amount needed in the body.

A. slightly in excess of
B. only a small percentage of
C. equal to
D. much in excess of

_A_   24.   Which of the following factors below does not explain the high incidence of osteoporosis in postmenopausal women?

A. Women have higher intakes of calcium than men.
B. Women are living longer today.
C. Weight reduction diets are common among women.
D. Lack of estrogen after menopause leads to bone loss.

_D_ 25. The mineral found in highest concentration in intracellular fluid (inside the cell) is:

    A. sodium. B. chloride. C. chromium. D. potassium.

_C_ 26. Edema represents:

    A. fluid loss from dehydration.
    B. too much base in body fluids.
    C. fluid in the extracellular space.
    D. too much acid in body fluids.

_D_ 27. Which of the following is the best food source of calcium?

    A. tomato juice B. butter C. spinach D. yogurt

_D_ 28. Significant food sources of potassium do not include:

    A. orange juice. B. dried fruits. C. bananas. D. cheese.

_C_ 29. Most water is lost daily via:

    A. the skin. B. the lungs. C. urine. D. feces.

_B_ 30. Most of the dietary phosphorus for Americans comes from:

    A. fruits and vegetables. C. whole grains.
    B. dairy products and meat. D. sugar and fat.

_B_ 31. In a comfortable environment water needs are about:

    A. 1 milliliter per pound of weight.
    B. 1 milliliter per kcalorie expended.
    C. 1 milliliter per square centimeter of body surface area.
    D. 1 milliliter per kilogram of body weight.

_B_ 32. Magnesium functions:

    A. in prevention of edema.
    B. as a cofactor in energy metabolism.
    C. as part of the thyroid hormone.
    D. in the transport of oxygen.

_D_ 33. Chloride:

    A. is the body's principal intracellular electrolyte.
    B. is necessary for protein synthesis in cells.
    C. protects bone structure against decalcification.
    D. helps maintain gastric acidity.

_B_ 34. Almost all (99%) of the calcium in the body is used to:

    A. maintain blood clotting.
    B. strengthen bones and teeth.
    C. provide energy for cells.
    D. regulate the transmission of nerve impulses.

_B_ 35. The calcium RDA for an adult over age 24 can essentially be met by consuming as part of an otherwise varied diet:

    A. 1 cup of spinach. C. 1 quart of milk.
    B. 2 cups of milk. D. a variety of plant foods.

Chapter 10
Weight Control

I.   Points to consider

Chapter 10 is designed to allow you to:

1.   Describe the uses of energy by the body and what constitutes energy balance.

2.   Outline physiological and environmental factors that influence food intake.

3.   Describe various ways of categorizing obesity.

4.   Outline the risks to health posed by obesity.

5.   List and discuss factors affecting energy balance in obesity, with respect to nature and nurture.

6.   Describe why and how reduced kcalorie intake, behavior modification, and increased physical activity fit into a weight loss plan.

7.   Outline the benefits and hazards of various weight-loss methods for severe (morbid) obesity.

8.   Evaluate fad weight reduction diets and determine which are unsafe, doomed to fail, or both.

II.   Word parts

Complete the following exercise using words in Chapter 10.

Word Part	Meaning	Examples
horm	impulse	__________
mes	middle	__________
morph	form, shape	__________
ba	stand	__________
therm	heat	__________
calor	heat	__________
plas	mold, shape	__________
morbid	characterized by disease	__________

III.   **Flash cards**

Cut out and review the flash cards for this chapter in Appendix A.

IV.   **Review and synthesis**

A.   1.   "In essence, hunger can be seen as our physiological drive to eat; appetite can be seen as our psychological drive to eat." Under each factor list two specific structures or mechanisms that influence us to begin eating or to end the process. (315)

<u>Hunger</u>   <u>Appetite</u>

Begin eating   a.   a.

                 b.   b.

Stop eating   a.   a.

                 b.   b.

2.   "I saw it, so I ate it." What drives your feeding behavior? List 3 possible factors and rank them according to the relative importance you think they have. (314)

a.

b.

c.

B.   "Energy used in basal metabolism depends primarily on lean body mass." Below are listed additional influences on basal metabolism. Explain briefly how each factor helps determine the metabolic rate (HINT: Does it increase it, decrease it, etc?). (316)

        a.   amount of body surface

        b.   gender

        c.   body temperature

        d.   thyroid hormone levels

        e.   age

        f.   nutritional state

        g.   pregnancy

        h.   caffeine and tobacco use

C.   "A predictable relationship exists between the body's use of energy and oxygen." Name and contrast the two methods of measuring energy use by the body. (319)

        a.

        b.

D.   1.   "Many health problems are caused by obesity." For the following health problems associated with excess body fat, list a possible reason why obesity can cause this health problem. (320)

<u>Health problem</u>   <u>Partially attributed to:</u>

Adult-onset diabetes mellitus
  (NIDDM)

Pulmonary disease

Hypertension

Coronary heart disease

Bone and joint disorders

Gallbladder stones

Various cancers

____

2.   "More than half of body fat lies directly under the skin." Describe two ways the amount
        of body fat can be estimated. (322)

        a.

        b.

3.   "Body weight is actually a crude measure, since we are concerned about overfat, not
        simply overweight individuals." Briefly describe three methods used to diagnose the
        extent of obesity. These also predict the degree of associated health risks. (321)

Degree of confidence	Method	Cutoff value
Rough estimate	a.	
	b.	
Sensitive estimate	c.	

E.   1.   "Evidence suggests that both nature and nurture influence the tendency for obesity."
             List three factors that tend to increase the risk of obesity. Classify each as primarily
             "nature" or "nurture". (329)

             a.

             b.

             c.

2.   "It is important for everyone to try to determine their own risk for obesity." State three reasons why adult-onset obesity could possibly develop in your adult years. (329)

    a.

    b.

    c.

F.   "They can be nurtured into gaining weight, allowing their natural tendency for obesity to blossom." Complete this table for a hamburger, a regular serving of french fries, and a strawberry milkshake. Recall the "4-4-9" relationship. Do the totals surprise you? (329)

	Protein (grams)	Carbohydrate (grams)	Fat (grams)	Kcalories
Quarter Pounder	25	29	24	_______
French fries	3	26	12	_______
Milk shake	9	62	9	_______
Totals:	_______	_______	_______	_______

G.   1.   "A sound weight loss program addresses the three key issues we have stressed." What three components provide the best approach to weight reduction? (332)

    a.

    b.

    c.

2.	List the two criteria that indicate weight loss has been successful. (330)

a.

b.

H.	"Without a strong behavioral plan, a lapse frequently turns into a relapse." List some techniques that help apply behavioral principles to a weight-loss plan. (335)

1.	Stimulus control

a. Shopping

b. Meal plans

c. Activities

d. Holidays and Parties

2.	Eating behavior

3.	Reward

4.	Self-monitoring

5.	Physical activity

a. Routine activity

b. Exercise

6.   Cognitive restructuring

7.   Contingency management

I.   "Exercise improves any diet." What are three benefits of increased physical activity in a weight-loss program? (337)

        a.

        b.

        c.

J.   "Muscle and other tissues generate the carbons used to make new glucose." Describe why initial weight loss can be so rapid on a low-carbohydrate diet. (340)

K.   "Underweight people should replace such foods as diet soft drinks with good energy sources, like fruit juices." List three practices a person could follow to gain weight. (341)

        a.

        b.

        c.

V.   **Applying nutrition to your life**

Choose a "diet" advertisement or article from a newspaper or magazine.

1.   List two statements in the article that force you to question the worth of the plan.

        a.

        b.

2.   Does your article cite an authority? If so, whom?

3.   What credentials are given for this authority?

4.   Overall, is the information in your article reliable? To what extent is it based on testimonials or unsubstantiated claims?

5.   Consider these potential characteristics for the diet advice. Answer yes or no in the space provided.

        a. Is it nutritionally balanced? _______

        b. Will kcalories actually be reduced? _______

        c. Does it provide for a variety of typical foods? _______

        d. Is it economical? _______

        e. Will it teach new eating habits? _______

        f. Can it be followed with modifications after weight is lost? _______

6.   Note any hazards or ill effects that might result from this particular diet.

VI.   Chapter 10 summary

Fill in the blanks using the words listed at the end of this summary.

Hunger, the _________ or __________ drive to find and eat food, is triggered partly by cells that form satiety and feeding centers in the _________. Destroy the satiety center in animals or humans and _________ with eventual obesity results. Destroy the feeding centers and _________ results. These centers monitor and respond to _________ and other nutrients. _________ and other compounds made by cells also help regulate body weight.

_________, the psychological desire to find and eat food, is affected by time of day, food availability and palatability, and _________. Because food is so readily available in the United States, appetite, not _________, is often the catalyst for food intake.

To some extent, body weight tends to regulate itself naturally. Does a "set point" for weight level exist? Trusting a set point to maintain a desirable weight isn't reliable; adults tend to gain ____ pounds between the ages of 18 and 54.

Basal metabolism, the thermic effect of food, and __________ account for most of the body's energy use. __________, the minimum energy needed to keep the resting body alive, is primarily determined by __________, amount of body surface, and thyroid hormone levels. The __________ of food is energy the body uses to digest, absorb, and process nutrients recently consumed. _______ energy taken in is stored as fat.

We measure the body's energy use directly, from _________, or indirectly, from __________. Formulas based on various combinations of body weight, height, and age estimate the body's energy needs.

Obesity can be defined along several dimensions:

1.   a total body fat exceeding __________ in men and 30% in women. Body fat is most often measured by ___________.

2.   a body mass index value (weight in kilograms divided by height in meters squared) over about _______.

3.	weighing _______ more than desirable body weight (based on the Metropolitan Life

	Insurance Table, published in 1983).

Fat distribution predicts health risks linked to obesity. _________ body fat storage (characterized

by a large abdomen and small buttocks and thighs) means higher risks of hypertension, heart disease,

and diabetes mellitus than with lower body obesity (small abdomen and larger buttocks and thighs).

_______ factors influence basal metabolism and body shape, and so influence the tendency to

obesity. How one is raised (or nurtured) also influences obesity, since _________ often develop similar

eating habits and activity patterns. Obesity may essentially be nurture allowing nature to be expressed.

When considering a treatment for obesity, remember (1) the body _______ weight loss; (2)

since obesity is difficult to reverse, the goal is ________; (3) lose weight mostly from _________, not

mostly from muscle and other lean tissues.

A ________ weight-loss diet should meet a dieter's nutritional needs by following the Food

Guide Pyramid. A good plan should adapt to the person's _________, encourage readily obtainable

foods, strive to change poor eating habits, promote regular _________ activity, and foster a lifelong

commitment to treatment. It should also insist that the dieter see a physician if weight is to be lost

_________ or if the person is over 35 years of age and plans to perform substantially greater physical

activity than usual.

A pound of fat tissue--gained or lost--represents approximately ________ kcalories. If energy

output _________ energy intake by 400 to 500 kcalories per day, one can lose a pound of fat storage in

a week. We can best cut kcalories by decreasing _________ foods.

_________ helps weight-loss programs because present habits may encourage overeating, and

discourage weight maintenance. Specific behavior modification techniques, such as _________ and

self-monitoring, help change problem behaviors.

Increasing physical activity sheds pounds. A good goal is to expend an extra _________

kcalories in activity each day.

Severe (morbid) obesity, defined as weighing at least _________ pounds over desirable body weight or twice the desirable body weight, may require (1) _________ surgery to reduce stomach volume to approximately 50 milliliters, or (2) very low calorie diets, containing 400 to 700 kcalories per day. Only people who _______ at more conservative approaches to weight loss should use these procedures.

Over-the-counter weight-loss medications include _________, other mild stimulants, and fiber pills. None of these, however, replace a good diet, behavior changes, and physical activity.

_________ probably make more unreasonable unproven and dangerous claims for fat ____________ treatments than for any other products. So-called ____________ show up everywhere -- television, ____________, and newspapers. The ancient advice still applies: "Let the buyer ____________." Some common characteristics of _________ diets are (1) they promote ____________ weight loss but little ___________ loss takes place and (2) they limit food ___________ and dictate specific ________.

Use the following words to complete the summary

	hormones	selections
appetite	hunger	semistarvation
basal metabolism	hypothalamus	skinfold thickness
behavior modification	internal	social custom
beware	lean body mass	sound
blood glucose	loss	stimulus control
cures	magazines	stomach
diet quacks	overeating	thermic effect
exceeds	oxygen uptake	unused
fad	phenylpropanolamine	upper
fail	physical	15 to 20
fat	physical activity	20%
fat storage	physiological	25%
family members	prevention	25-27
genetic	quick	100
habits	rapidly	200 to 300
heat output	resists	2700
high fat	rituals	

Check your answers using the summary for Chapter 10 in your textbook and page 130 of this <u>Study Guide</u> for the last nine answers.

   Practice examination.

Cover the answers for your initial attempt.

__B__   1.   Decreasing kcalorie intake by 400-500 kcalories per day would mean a loss of about one pound of body fat in:

   A. 2 days.
   B. 7 days.
   C. 10 days.
   D. 14 days.

__C__   2.   If remaining at rest, an adult would use about how many kcalories in a day?

   A. 500   B. 800   C. 1400   D. 2500

__D__   3.   Diet-induced thermogenesis represents the energy cost of:

   A. chewing food.
   B. peristalsis.
   C. basal metabolism.
   D. digesting, absorbing, and packaging nutrients.

__C__   4.   A significant health hazard from obesity is:

   A. ulcers.
   B. diverticulosis.
   C. diabetes mellitus.
   D. emphysema.

For questions 5 to 12 indicate the effect of each of the following conditions on basal metabolism. (You may use A, B, and C more than once.)

   A. increases it   B. decreases it   C. has no effect

__A__   5.   more lean body mass
__A__   6.   fever
__B__   7.   fasting
__A__   8.   pregnancy
__A__   9.   large body surface area
__C__   10.   mental thought
__B__   11.   weight loss diet
__B__   12.   aging

__C__   13.   The hypothalamus:

   A. increases metabolism for more efficient use of energy.
   B. drives the psychological need for hunger.
   C. contains a regulatory feeding center.
   D. stops working after age 65.

__C__   14.   A hormone involved in regulating basal metabolism is:

   A. insulin.
   B. gastrin.
   C. thyroxine.
   D. glucagon.

__B__   15.   What percentage of a day's total caloric need is used for digesting, absorbing, transporting, and storing nutrients (the thermic effect of food)?

   A. 1% to 3%
   B. 5% to 10%
   C. 15% to 20%
   D. 25% to 30%

__C__   16.   What body fat concentration is the cutoff for obesity in men?

   A. 10%   B. 15%   C. 25%   D. 30%

| D | 17. | An example of a behavior modification technique for weight control is: |

A. always clean your plate when you eat.
B. have someone criticize you if you overeat.
C. feel guilty after you overeat.
D. keep a record of your eating habits so you can see what situations cause you
to overeat.

| C | 18. | To lose 1 pound of body weight in a week, a person would have to reduce daily kcalories by: |

A. 50 to 100.   D. 1000 to 1100.
B. 150 to 250.   E. 2700 to 3500.
C. 400 to 500.

| D | 19. | Probably the most important reason for obesity today in the United States is: |

A. the set-point theory.   C. "eating on the run".
B. genetic selection.   D. inactivity.

| D | 20. | Problems encountered with the use of drugs to lose weight include: |

A. drugs may produce serious side effects.
B. many drugs induce the loss of body fluid, but not body fat.
C. drugs do not lead to permanent changes in eating habits.
D. all of the above.

| B | 21. | A general weight reduction diet should contain no less than: |

A. 600 to 800 kcalories per day.
B. 1000 to 1200 kcalories per day.
C. 1500 to 1800 kcalories per day.
D. 2000 to 2200 kcalories per day.

| A | 22. | People on weight reduction diets should avoid: |

A. high-fat foods.
B. breads and rolls.
C. potatoes.
D. meat.

| D | 23. | A weight reduction program can be considered successful only when the weight loss: |

A. is done without harming one's health.
B. is maintained permanently.
C. includes loss of body fat, body protein, and body water.
D. A and B

| A | 24. | The best approach for weight loss is to: |

A. reduce daily energy intake and increase energy expenditure.
B. avoid foods containing carbohydrates.
C. greatly increase protein intake to prevent body protein loss.
D. cut down on water intake.

| C | 25. | What is usually the major factor that explains variability in the kcalorie needs of two healthy men of similar age and size? |

A. brown adipose tissue metabolism
B. basal metabolism
C. physical activity
D. type of diet consumed

  C   26.   Which of the following foods often is high in fat?

                A. 1% milk
                B. bread
                C. meat
                D. green vegetables
                E. fruits

  B   27.   A reasonable weight-loss goal is:

                A. no more than 1/4 pound per week.
                B. 1 to 2 pounds per week.
                C. 5 to 6 pounds per week.
                D. depends on one's dominant gland.

  D   28.   A low-carbohydrate diet causes:

                A. an increase in extracellular fluid.
                B. glycogen synthesis.
                C. increased rate of normal metabolism.
                D. use of muscle tissue to produce glucose.

  A   29.   The most effective treatment for obesity is:

                A. a kcalorie intake less than kcalorie output.
                B. diuretic therapy.
                C. use of hormones to increase basal metabolism.
                D. a high-protein diet.

  B   30.   A major weakness of a low fat diet is:

                A. essential fatty acid deficiency.
                B. relative lack of satiety.
                C. too little fiber.
                D. too much linoleic acid.

  C   31.   When using physical activity to help lose weight, the key is:

                A. intensity.
                B. improving sports skills.
                C. duration and regularity.
                D. doing it at 6 AM.

  A   32.   Initial weight loss on a fad diet is often:

                A. water, glycogen, and lean tissue.
                B. abdominal fat.
                C. sex-specific fat.
                D. edema.

  B   33.   Behavior modification in obesity treatment includes:

                A. following the physician's orders to the letter.
                B. understanding and correcting poor dietary habits.
                C. very low kcalorie diets.
                D. gastric bypass surgery.

_A_   34.   The intent of gastroplasty (stomach stapling) is to:

A. limit stomach volume.
B. speed transit time.
C. limit ability for absorption.
D. prevent snacking.

Answers to selected questions

VI. diet quacks, loss, cures, magazines, beware, fad, quick, fat, selections, rituals

---

Chapter 11
Nutrition: Athletics and Fitness

I.   **Points to consider**

Chapter 11 is designed to allow you to:

1.   Define metabolism and explain what is meant by anabolic and catabolic pathways.

2.   Identify the major sources of energy for the body and illustrate various ways cells obtain ATP energy.

3.   Show an understanding of glycolysis, differentiating between aerobic and anaerobic metabolism.

4.   Describe the various energy systems used by muscles and when each is used by the muscle.

5.   Examine the importance of carbohydrate in an athlete's diet and the importance of carbohydrate intake to athletic training.

6.   Show an understanding of the importance of maintaining stores of various vitamins and minerals during exercise.

7.   Outline the importance of water, sports drinks or both during exercise.

8.   Define ergogenic aids and describe their effects on an athlete's performance.

9.   Identify how regular physical activity can have a beneficial effect on the body.

II.   **Word parts**

Complete the following exercise using words in Chapter 11.

Word Part	Meaning	Examples
metabo	change	__________
anabo	to build up	__________
catabo	breakdown	__________
tri	three	__________
di	two	__________
post	after	__________
glyco	sugar	__________

III.   **Flash cards**

Cut out and review the flash cards for this chapter in Appendix A.

IV.   **Review and synthesis**

A.   1.   "Essentlally, adenosine triphosphate (ATP) is the immediate source of energy for body functions." Briefly define ATP and describe the process of how ATP is formed. (354)

         2.   "Carbohydrates are a valuable fuel for muscles. The most useful form of carbohydrate fuel is the simple sugar glucose." Illustrate the basic process of glycolysis and explain the difference between its two pathways--aerobic and anaerobic. (356)

B.   "The main advantages of PCr is that it can be activated instantly and can replenish ATP at rates fast enough to meet the energy demands of the fastest and most powerful sports events, including jumping, lifting, throwing, and sprinting actions." Table 11-1 describes several energy systems used by muscle cells. Complete the following table, indicating when various energy sources are used and give one example of an exercise. (356)

<u>System</u>	<u>When in use</u>	<u>Examples of an exercise</u>
ATP		
phosphocreatine		
anaerobic glycolysis		
aerobic glycolysis		
aerobic fat utilization		
aerobic protein utilization		

C.   "Anyone who exercises regularly, including the dieter, needs to consume a diet that includes moderate to high amounts of carbohydrates." Use Tables 11-3 and 11-4 to design a day's meal pattern that is high in carbohydrates. First convert 55% of total kcalories to grams of carbohydrates. If you are male, base 55% on a 3000-kcalorie diet; if you are female, use a 2500-kcalorie diet. Add up the number of grams as carbohydrates in each food choice. Does it exceed the number of grams you calculated as a goal? (365)

2.   "It is often advantageous to undertake a carbohydrate-loading regimen to maximize muscle glycogen stores." Briefly describe carbohydrate loading: the process, what is the expected result, and a potential disadvantage. (364)

3.   "High carbohydrate foods should be emphasized, and should dominate the pre-event meal." Give an example of a pre- and post-event meal, including when the meal should be eaten. (369)

Pre-event meal	Activity	Post-event meal
Time:	Time:	Time:

D.   "During muscle-building regimens, athletes should consume 1 to 1.5 grams of protein per kilogram of body weight every day." (367) First calculate the number of grams of protein you would need (recall 2.2 pounds = 1 kilogram). Then indicate several protein-containing foods that would meet this requirement." (See Figure 7-7 or Appendix A in your textbook for excellent protein sources.)

E.   "Athletes should pay very close attention to their vitamin and mineral intake." Review the advice provided for athletes for both iron and calcium intake in the textbook. Highlight some major points below. (367)

Iron:

Calcium:

F.   "Athletes need enough water to maintain the body's ability to regulate its internal temperature and so keep itself cool." Outline how sweating regulates body temperature and why fluid replacement is necessary. (369)

What is the general rule for timing and amount of fluid replacement?

V.   Applying nutrition to your life

"Even a minimal amount of exercise--a brisk half-hour walk a few times a week--is important for promoting fitness. Overall, exercise should be a regular part of one's life." (361) A basic exercise program should consist of a warm-up exercise, an exercise to increase muscular strength, endurance and flexibility, and finally a cool-down exercise. Design your own exercise program for one week. Include warm-up (stretching), exercise activity and length of the exercise, measure of heart rate, and cool-down exercise. Now track your exercise and related fluid intake for the next week.

<u>Warm-up and Cool-down</u>

Monday

Tuesday

Wednesday

Thursday

Friday

Saturday

Sunday

<u>Activity</u>	<u>Typical heart rate</u>	<u>Time exercised</u>	<u>Fluid intake (cups)</u>
Monday			
Tuesday			
Wednesday			
Thursday			
Friday			
Saturday			
Sunday			
Average heart rate (total/7) _________	Average time (total/7) _________	Average cups (total/7) _________	

How much total water or fluid did you generally drink--before, after, and during exercise? Was this enough fluid to minimize fatigue and keep body weight constant?

VI.   Chapter 11 summary

Fill in the blanks using the words listed at the end of this summary.

______________ is the major form of energy for cellular metabolism. As ATP is breaking down into ADP plus a ______________ group, energy is released. All energy available to humans comes from ______________ energy. Plants capture solar energy using ______________. Human metabolic pathways are able to extract that energy from foodstuffs and ______________ it into ATP energy. ______________ can also provide the energy needed to reform ATP.

In ______________, glucose is broken down into a 3-carbon compound, yielding in addition some ATP. The 3-carbon compound can then proceed to other ______________ pathways to form carbon dioxide and ______________, or anaerobic pathways to form ______________ acid.

At low workload, muscle cells mostly use ______________ for fuel. For intense exercise of short duration, muscles use the ______________ for energy. For more sustained intense activity, muscle glycogen breaks down and enters the ______________ pathway, forming lactic acid. For endurance exercise, fat and carbohydrates are used as ______________. Carbohydrates are used increasingly as activity intensifies. Little ______________ is used to fuel muscles.

______________ is a vital part of a healthy lifestyle. Stretching exercises and aerobic stimulation of the ______________ should be a goal of any exercise plan. Physically active people show lower risks for heart disease, ______________, and other common chronic diseases.

Anyone who exercises needs to consume a diet that is moderate to high in ______________ and which follows the suggestions of the ______________. Vitamin and mineral supplements are indicated when ______________ energy intakes make it difficult to ______________ needs. Carbohydrate loading can ______________ the usual stores of muscle ______________. Participants in endurance events lasting more than ______________ hours can benefit most from carbohydrate loading. This utilizes a diet containing about ______________ grams of carbohydrate for 3 to 4 days before the event. Athletes should consume enough ______________ to maintain body weight during exercise. A ______________ drink can be helpful for endurance athletes. __________ aids are thought to enhance __________. Proven aids include carbohydrate and water,

__________ as well as __________ in some sporting events.

Use the following words to complete the summary

aerobic	fluid	phosphate
ATP	fuels	photosynthesis
caffeine	glycogen	protein
carbohydrate	glycolysis	sports type
convert	glycolytic	solar
Guide to Daily Food Choices	heart	water
diabetes	lactic	2
double	low nutrient	600
ergogenic	performance	
exercise	phosphocreatine	
fat	phosphocreatine system	

Check your answers using the summary for Chapter 11 in your textbook.

VII.   Practice examination

Cover the answers on your initial attempt.

__B__   1.   The process in which plants use solar energy to produce carbohydrates is known as:

    A. glycolysis.   C. the Krebs cycle.
    B. photosynthesis.   D. none of the above.

__D__   2.   The special form of energy used by cells is called:

    A. ADP.   C. glucose.
    B. phosphocreatine.   D. ATP.

__B__   3.   When glucose is broken down in an atmosphere where oxygen supply is limited, a 3-carbon component known as ___________________ accumulates in the muscle.

    A. glycogen   C. phosphocreatine
    B. lactic acid   D. nitrogen

__C__   4.   When there is plenty of oxygen available in the muscles, the condition is referred to as being:

    A. anaerobic.   C. aerobic.
    B. oxygenated.   D. ventilated.

__A__   5.   What is the major disadvantage of accumulating lactic acid in the muscles?

    A. fatigue.   C. nausea.
    B. muscle damage.   D. none - it's an advantage.

__B__   6.   What is the preferable fuel for anaerobic glycolysis in an activity lasting less than two hours?

    A. fatty acid   C. glucose
    B. glycogen   D. amino acids

137

| C | 7. | . Athletes often take carnitine pills in order to ________________. However, this is of no value. |

A. provide glycogen stones   C. burn fat faster
B. build muscles   D. increase foot speed

| B | 8. | What source of energy is mainly used in light, aerobic activity? |

A. carbohydrate   C. protein
B. fat   D. all of the above

| D | 9. | Which of the foods below constitutes the best choice when one attempts carbohydrate loading before endurance events? |

A. potato chips   C. all bran (high-fiber) cereal
B. french fries   D. rice

| C | 10. | During muscle building regimens, athletes should consume how many grams of protein per kilogram of body weight? |

A. 0.5 to 0.7 grams per kilograms.   C. 1 to 1.5 grams per kilograms.
B. 0.8 grams per kilograms.   D. 2 grams per kilograms.

| B | 11. | During training the recommended dietary allowances for vitamins are greatly increased. |

A. True   B. False

| D | 12. | It is a good idea, especially for adult women athletes, to have blood hemoglobin levels regularly checked for deficiencies of what mineral? |

A. calcium   C. copper
B. potassium   D. iron

| C | 13. | There has recently been found a correlation between low density of spinal bone in women and: |

A. type of exercise.   C. lack of menstruation.
B. weight.   D. iron deficiency.

| C | 14. | A light meal is best eaten ____________ hours before a sporting event? |

A. 4 to 6 hours   C. 2 to 4 hours
B. immediately before to   D. you should not eat on the
    give a boost of energy   day of a sports event

| C | 15. | Caffeine, along with ________________, has a dehydrating effect on the body, so fluids containing them should not be part of any hydration plan for exercise. |

A. sugared soft drinks   C. alcohol
B. dairy products   D. carbohydrate solutions

| D | 16. | Which of the following items is considered to be the best ergogenic aid to increase athletic performance? |

A. bee pollen   C. coenzyme Q 10
B. salt tablets   D. none of the above

| B | 17. | An ergogenic aid that is used in order to control lactic acid buildup in muscle is: |

A. caffeine.   C. anabolic steroid.
B. bicarbonate.   D. growth hormone.

Chapter 12
Anorexia Nervosa and Bulimia

I.   **Points to consider**

Chapter 12 is designed to allow you to:

1. Contrast healthy attitudes toward uses of food with behavior patterns that could lead to unhealthy uses of food.

2. Outline the causes of, effects of, typical persons affected by, and treatment for anorexia nervosa.

3. Outline the causes of, effects of, typical persons affected by, and treatment for bulimia.

4. Outline the causes of, effects of, typical persons affected by, and treatment for compulsive eating.

5. Relate the existence of eating disorders to current social trends.

6. Describe methods to reduce the development of eating disorders, including the use of early warning signs to identify early cases.

II.   **Word parts**

Complete the following exercise using words in Chapter 12.

Word Part	Meaning	Examples
or	mouth	_______________
lim	hunger	_______________
kal	potassium	_______________
bar	weight	_______________
lan	wool	_______________
syn	with, together	_______________
bary	heavy	_______________

III.   **Flash cards**

Cut out and review the flash cards for this chapter in Appendix A.

IV.   Review and synthesis

A.   "Everyday we are bombarded with images of the 'ideal' body. Television programs, billboard advertisements, magazine pictures, movies and newspapers tell us that an ultra-slim body will bring happiness, love, and even success." (382)

1.   Name two media examples that influenced you to think or act in a different way, and how, if taken to the extreme, these influences could be destructive.

a.

b.

2.   Name three constructive and healthy ways (related to food) that you personally can work toward a happy, successful life.

a.

b.

c.

B.   "The only thing I am good at is dieting. I can't do anything else." Complete the following table. Keep in mind these eating disorders often overlap, but ignore that for now. (384)

	Societal pressures that may trigger disease	Physical signs and symptom	Psychological straits
Anorexia nervosa			
Bulimia			

C.	"A person with anorexia nervosa refuses to eat. That behavior is the hallmark of the disease, whether or not other practices such as binge-purge cycles appear." Sally is a 19-year old college sophomore with a 7-year history of anorexia nervosa. She is 5 feet, 7 inches tall and weighs 90 pounds. List six of the possible physical effects of anorexia nervosa on her. (386)

a.

b.

c.

d.

e.

f.

D.	1.	"Susceptible people may have both biological factors and lifestyle patterns that predispose them to becoming overweight." From what you know about the physiology and characteristics of obesity, describe three possible predisposing factors for bulimia. (390)

a.

b.

c.

	2.	Add to this list three societal factors that can increase the risk for development of bulimia. (390)

a.

b.

c.

E.   "The major difference from anorexia nervosa is that the bulimic person turns to food during a crisis or problem, not away from it." Do your life situations affect your response to food, causing you to eat either more or less than usual? Name three alternative coping mechanisms you could use at these times (consult Chapter 10 if needed). (393)

a.

b.

c.

F.   "Among sufferers of bulimia, binges often alternate with attempts to rigidly restrict food intake." Explain the process (or cycle) of bingeing and purging. (391)

G.   "Compulsive overeating can be viewed as eating to avoid feeling and dealing with emotional pain." Although it is also classified as an eating disorder, how does compulsive overeating in general differ from bulimia and anorexia nervosa? (394)

What are two ways compulsive overeaters can help overcome their disorder?

a.

b.

V.   Applying nutrition to your life

"One of your best friends may practice bulimia without your knowing it. The person may feel desperate, yet will go to great lengths to keep it secret." You suspect that your roommate, close friend, or spouse practices bulimia.

1.   How might you approach that person with your concerns?

2.   What steps could you take to aid that person in getting professional help and during treatment?

3.   Who else can help you with this situation? Why?

4.   Is there any place on your campus or in the surrounding community where a person can receive help with an eating disorder? If yes, where is it located? If no, investigate further, since most communities have these resources.

VI.   Chapter 12 summary

Fill in the blanks using the words listed at the end of this summary.

The person with anorexia nervosa is usually a girl around the age of ________ who begins to

diet, but then finds it difficult to stop. The person is generally a _________ and high achiever, often

described as the "best little girl in the world." Few cases are seen in ___________. Warning signs for

anorexia nervosa include abnormal food habits, such as cutting a pea in half before eating it or cooking a large meal and _____________ others eat. Later, _______ performance crumbles, the person often refuses to eat out with family and friends, and she develops a very ________ and joyless nature.

Physical effects of anorexia nervosa include a decrease in body temperature, and in _______ iron deficiency _______, a low white blood cell count, hair loss, constipation, a low blood _________ level, and the loss of ___________. Treatment of anorexia nervosa includes increasing food intake to at least a level sufficient to support _________, and then to allow for gradual weight gain. Psychological counseling attempts to help the person establish ______ food habits and to find means of coping with the _________ that led to the disorder. _________ may be necessary. Bulimia is characterized by _________ on up to 20,000 kcalories at one sitting, and then _________ by _________, _________ use, exercise, or other means. Both men and women are at risk. Vomiting as a means of purging is especially destructive to the body: it can cause severe _________, stomach ulcers, irritation of the esophagus, low blood potassium levels, and other problems. Bulimia poses a serious health problem and is associated with significant risk of _______.

Treatment of bulimia includes ____________, as well as nutritional counseling. During treatment, the person learns to ____________ himself or herself and to cope with problems in ways which do not involve ____________. Regular ____________ patterns are developed as the bulimic person begins to plan meals in an informed, ____________ manner.

____________ describes a condition where children are ____________ by parents in an attempt to limit risk of future disease, such as _______________ or heart disease. Growth failure -- reduced weight and height gains -- can result if ____________ intake is not increased to appropriate levels.

_________ and food binges not associated with purging are two behaviors characteristic of _________. Emotional disturbances are often at the root of this disordered form of eating. Treatment addresses deeper _________, avoidance of _________ and _________, and restoration of normal eating behaviors.

____________ has been ranked as the most dreaded deviation from our cultural ideals of body image. Over the course of this century, a woman's "ideal" body form has become ____________.

Researchers have linked this preference for a ______________ body type to the recent surge in

______________________.

Use the following words to complete the summary

accept	fatness	men	regular
anemia	food	menstrual periods	restrictive diets
baryophobia	food deprivation	nutrient	school
basal metabolism	grazing	obesity	suicide
bingeing	healthy	perfectionist	thinner
compulsive	heart rate	potassium	tooth decay
overeating	hospitalization	psychological	underfed
critical	laxative	puberty	vomiting
eating	lean	purging	watching
eating disorders	life stresses		
emotional issues			

Check your answers using the summary for Chapter 12 in your textbook and page 146 of this <u>Study Guide</u> for the last nine answers.

VII. Practice examination
Cover the answers on your initial attempt.

___A___ 1. A long-term health consequence of anorexia nervosa could be:

     A. fractures resulting in bone loss.   C. infertility.
     B. atherosclerotic heart disease.   D. cancer.

___B___ 2. An early warning sign of anorexia nervosa is:

     A. hoarding food.   C. secret bingeing.
     B. withdrawal from family.   D. use of ipecac syrup.

___A___ 3. The major health risk from frequent vomiting due to bulimia is:

     A. a potassium imbalance.   C. lanugo.
     B. constipation.   D. swollen glands.

For questions 4 to 13 indicate which of the following characteristics are mainly associated with anorexia nervosa (A), and which are mainly associated with bulimia (B). Ignore that some characteristics may be associated with both eating disorders.

___A___ 4. Intense fear of becoming obese.

___B___ 5. Aware of abnormal eating pattern.

___A___ 6. Distorted image of body size.

___B___ 7. Depressed mood following binges.

___B___ 8. May be above desirable weight for height.

___A___ 9. Fear of not being able to stop eating.

___A___ 10. Loss of menses.

| A | 11. | Refusal to maintain body weight within normal limits. |

| B | 12. | Secretive eating. |

| A | 13. | Compulsive physical activity. |

| C | 14. | Which of the following does <u>not</u> describe people suffering from starvation? |

    A. state of extreme weakness and collapse
    B. mental disorientation
    C. hyperactive, hungry, and actively clamoring for food
    D. extreme apathy and indifference

| D | 15. | Anorexia nervosa is a disease of: |

    A. children.   C. young boys.
    B. elderly women.   D. teenage women.

| C | 16. | The most successful treatment for anorexia nervosa involves: |

    A. isolation from the family and forced tube feeding.
    B. dietary counseling on an outpatient basis by a registered dietitian.
    C. inpatient psychological, nutritional, and medical therapy, often involving the whole family.
    D. use of diuretics.

| C | 17. | A critical goal in the early stages of the treatment of a person with anorexia is to: |

    A. increase the patient's weight to her goal body weight within the first month.
    B. establish regular meal patterns.
    C. allow the person a feeling of control over her life.
    D. get the patient to realize how unbecoming her body has become.

| D | 18. | Bulimic patients often have a problem with: |

    A. recognizing nutritious food choices.
    B. eating enough food to maintain a healthy body weight.
    C. obesity.
    D. an inability to control responses to impulse and desire.

| B | 19. | Characteristics of a person exhibiting compulsive overeating often include: |

    A. a persistent concern with body shape, weight, and thinness.
    B. regularly eating to avoid feeling and dealing with emotional pain.
    C. family history with a constrictive internal structure.
    D. adoption of rigid "food rules".

| D | 20. | For a person with compulsive overeating, food is used to: |

    A. reduce stress and avoid life problems.
    B. produce feelings of power and well-being.
    C. avoid feelings of intimacy with others.
    D. all of the above.

Answers to selected questions

VI. fatness; thinner; lean; eating disorders; grazing; compulsive overeating; emotional issues; food deprivation; restrictive diets

---

Chapter 13
Pregnancy and Breast-feeding

I.   **Points to consider**

Chapter 13 is designed to allow you to:

1. List major changes occurring in the body during pregnancy and the altered nutrient needs associated with each change.

2. List factors that may interfere with a successful pregnancy outcome.

3. Specify the optimal weight gain during pregnancy for the normal adult woman.

4. Plan an adequate, balanced diet for the pregnant woman and the breast-feeding woman using the Food Guide Pyramid as a basis.

5. Identify the nutrients that may need to be supplemented during pregnancy and explain the reason for each.

6. Explain how typical discomforts of pregnancy may be minimized by diet changes.

7. Describe the physiology of breast-feeding and give some advantages of breast-feeding for the mother and infant.

II.   **Word parts**

Complete the following exercise using words in Chapter 13.

Word Part	Meaning	Examples
nat	to be born	__________
gest	to bear	__________
fet	offspring	__________
pica	magpie	__________
tri	three	__________
syn	together, with	__________

III. Flash cards

Cut out and review the flash cards for this chapter in Appendix A.

IV.   **Review and synthesis**

A.   "Education, an adequate diet, and early and consistent prenatal medical care maximize the chances of producing a healthy baby." List three problems that may contribute to a higher risk during pregnancy. Briefly outline the mechanism for each. (423)

    a.

    b.

    c.

B.   "The RDA for protein increases by 10 grams daily." The fetus needs nutrients for energy and for the growth and development of tissues and organs. List two key nutrients associated with each of the following. Then list a good food source for each. (420)

Increased Need	Key Nutrient	Food Source
a. Protein synthesis	_________	_________
	_________	_________
b. Bone growth	_________	_________
	_________	_________
c. Energy metabolism	_________	_________
	_________	_________
d. Collagen formation	_________	_________
	_________	_________
e. Blood formation	_________	_________
	_________	_________

Check your answers using page 158 of this <u>Study Guide</u>.

C.	"In addition, researchers in Great Britain showed that height and social class could better predict the outcome of pregnancy than dietary intake during pregnancy." What are two possible consequences if a woman enters pregnancy in poor nutritional status? Postulate a reason for each. (422)

a.

b.

D.	"Nutrient needs for a breast-feeding mother change slightly -- if at all -- from those of the pregnant woman." (432) Compare the RDA for the following nutrients for a pregnant woman with those for a lactating woman. (Use the inside cover of your textbook.)

NUTRIENT	A.Pregnant woman	B.Lactating woman	Difference (A - B)	Food Choice	Amount of the nutrient present
Protein					
Vitamin A					
Vitamin D					
Thiamin					
Riboflavin					
Niacin					
Vitamin C					
Calcium					
Zinc					

Use Appendix A in your textbook to check if the nutrient content of the potential food choices supply the increased needs you listed. See if just one or two food choices will suffice to meet all extra nutrient needs.

E. "As stated earlier the Food Guide Pyramid provides a good diet approach during pregnancy."
Outline the diet plan for pregnant women proposed in your textbook. Indicate approximate
serving sizes. (420)

Food group	Number of servings
Milk, yogurt, and cheese	
Meat, poultry, fish, dry beans, eggs, and nuts	
Vegetables	
Fruits	
Breads, cereals, rice, and pasta	

F. "She cannot afford a 'Big Mac' for herself and another for the fetus." In what way must a
pregnant woman eat for two? Why? (414)

G. "Maternal dietary changes during pregnancy will enable the typical woman to meet all increased
needs for nutrients, except perhaps for iron." What two nutrients are the focus of
supplementation in the diet during pregnancy? Why? (420)

a.

b.

H.   "A total vegetarian (vegan) must carefully plan a diet for pregnancy." List four nutrient needs the pregnant vegan should pay special attention to. Indicate a food source for each. (421)

a.

b.

c.

d.

I.   "Although a mother's digestive and metabolic systems work very efficiently, some discomfort accompanies the changes her body undergoes to accommodate the fetus." List four common complaints of pregnancy that may be related to diet. Briefly indicate how to try to solve each problem. (427)

a.

b.

c.

d.

J.   1.   "Human milk is tailored to meet infant nutrient needs for the first 4 to 6 months of life. The possible exceptions are fluoride, iron, and vitamin D." Compare and contrast use of human milk and commercial infant formulas. (433)

Factors	Human milk	Commercial formula
Prevention of infections		
Risk of contamination		
Risk of allergies		
Convenience		

---

2.   "Although formula feeding can satisfy the infant, breast-feeding offers many physiological advantages." Breast-feeding benefits both the mother and infant. What are three potential benefits not listed in Part 1 for either the mother or the infant? (434)

a.

b.

c.

V.   Applying nutrition to your life

A.   "Breast-feeding reduces the general risk of infections to the infant." If you were asked to conduct a class for pregnant women on the benefits of breast-feeding, what 4 main points would you highlight during this session? (433)

      a.

      b.

      c.

      d.

B.   How would you answer the following questions? (434)

      a.   How can I continue to breast-feed when I am at work?

      b.   Is it OK to have a glass of wine at dinner while I'm breast-feeding?

      c.   How old should my baby be when I begin to wean him or her from the breast?

      d.   Is it OK to diet while I'm breast-feeding?

      e.   How do I know if my infant is getting enough milk?

VI.   Chapter 13 summary

Fill in the blanks using the words listed at the end of this summary.

Adequate nutrition is vital during pregnancy to ensure the well-being of both the infant and the mother. Problems caused by poor nutrition and some medications can cause __________, and especially if this occurs in the first trimester. Growth retardation and altered development are possible if insults occur later in pregnancy. Infants born _________ (before 37 weeks of gestation) or with low ________ (less than 5.5 pounds, or 2500 grams) usually have more medical problems at birth than do normal infants. _______ pregnancy requires very careful prenatal and nutritional care. Complications occur more often in these pregnancies because of the very high ________ demands and often poor social and economic support.

Daily energy needs increase by an average of _______ kcalories during the last two trimesters of pregnancy. Weight gain should be gradual, reaching a total of ______ pounds in a normal-weight mother. Protein, vitamin, and mineral requirements increase with pregnancy. Extra servings from the __________ and the meat, poultry, fish and beans group of the Guide to Daily Food Choices are recommended. ________ and folate in particular may need to be supplemented in the diet. Pregnancy-induced hypertension, _______, constipation, nausea and vomiting, edema, and _______ are all possible discomforts and complications of pregnancy. Nutrition therapy can often help minimize these problems.

The popularity of breast-feeding has increased in the past 20 years. Almost all women have the ability to nurse their infants. The nutrient composition of human milk is very different from _________________. The first fluid called __________, is very rich in __________. Advantages of breast-feeding over formula-feeding include fewer infant intestinal, respiratory, and ear ________; fewer infant _______ and intolerances; and convenience. An infant can be adequately nourished with formula if the mother chooses not to breast-feed. Breast-feeding is not desirable if the mother has certain diseases or must take ________ that are potentially harmful to the infant.

__________ is one potential energy source that should be avoided during pregnancy. _________ are commonly seen in infants exposed to high amounts _________. More subtle defects in development are suspected at lower intakes.

Use the following words to complete the summary

alcohol	cow's milk	medications
allergies	heart burn	milk and cheese group
anemia	immune factors	physiological
birth defects	infection	prematurely
birth weight	in utero	teenage
colostrum	iron	24 to 28
		300

Check your answers using the summary for Chapter 13 in your textbook and page 158 of this <u>Study Guide</u> for the last two answers.

Cover the answers on your initial attempt.

D   1.   Which of the following mothers probably faces the highest pregnancy risk?

A. white, mature, lower socioeconomic family
B. adolescent, nonwhite, upper middle-class family
C. white, mature, middle-class family
D. adolescent, nonwhite, lower socioeconomic family

B   2.   The pregnant woman needs to increase her kcalorie intake by about ______ per day during the last two trimesters of pregnancy.

A. 100 kcalories   C. 500 kcalories
B. 300 kcalories   D. 800 kcalories

C   3.   The breast-feeding woman with normal fat stores from pregnancy needs to increase her kcalorie intake by about ______ per day.

A. 100 kcalories   C. 500 kcalories
B. 300 kcalories   D. 800 kcalories

D   4.   Which of the following is <u>not</u> an attribute of human milk?

A. lactose content
B. presence of a bifidus factor
C. antibody content
D. high mineral content

D   5.   The hormone responsible for the let-down reflex in breast-feeding is:

A. thyroid-stimulating hormone.   C. insulin.
B. prolactin.   D. oxytocin.

C   6.   Which of the following is <u>not</u> a component of weight gain in pregnancy?

A. breast tissue   C. thigh muscles
B. amniotic fluid   D. blood volume

D   7.   An energy source to avoid in pregnancy is:

A. fat.   C. carbohydrate.
B. protein.   D. alcohol.

B   8.   Weight gain in pregnancy should usually be at least about:

A. 16 pounds.   B. 25 pounds.   C. 30 pounds.   D. 36 pounds.

B   9.   A major advantage of breast-feeding for the infant is:

A. the <u>E. coli</u> factor.   C. the high casein content.
B. passive immunity.   D. low lactose content.

B   10.   Colostrum:

A. can be synthesized by the newborn infant, but not by a fetus.
B. is a source of antibodies and secreted for the first few days after birth.
C. contains mainly fat.
D. is a hormone involved in stimulating lactation.

| B | 11. | It is often recommended that breast-fed infants be supplemented with which of the following nutrients? |

A. iron and vitamin B-6
B. vitamin D and iron
C. calcium and iron
D. vitamin C and vitamin D

| C | 12. | The fetus receives nourishment primarily through: |

A. antibodies. C. the placenta.
B. meconium. D. amniotic fluid.

| B | 13. | During pregnancy the woman who is a vegan may not obtain adequate amounts of which of the following nutrients? |

A. niacin, vitamin D, magnesium, and iodide
B. calcium, iron, zinc, and vitamin B-12
C. thiamin, niacin, riboflavin, and folate
D. vitamin C, vitamin B-6, phosphorus, and sodium

| D | 14. | An attribute of human milk that keeps the infant from supporting the growth of some harmful intestinal bacteria is: |

A. lactase. C. let-down reflex.
B. albumin. D. bifidus factor.

| A | 15. | In general, nutritional deficits in the breast-feeding mother: |

A. reduce the quantity of her milk.
B. reduce all nutrients equally.
C. stop lactation entirely.
D. reduce the quality of her milk.

| C | 16. | The let-down reflex: |

A. causes depression in a new mother after the birth.
B. moves the hindmilk toward the nipple after the infant has drawn the foremilk.
C. forces milk to the nipple area of the breast.
D. makes a newborn turn toward whichever cheek is touched and search for the nipple.

| C | 17. | An increased requirement for _________ during pregnancy is related to their roles in the synthesis of red blood cells. |

A. vitamin E and vitamin C
B. iron and vitamin K
C. folate and vitamin B-12
D. protein and calcium

| A | 18. | The "physiological anemia of pregnancy" is a result of a(n): |

A. increase in the mother's blood volume.
B. decrease in the mother's iron absorption.
C. decrease in the mother's water consumption.
D. decrease in the mother's red blood cell production.

| D | 19. | A maternal practice that can be harmful to the fetus is: |

A. a low-carbohydrate diet. C. smoking.
B. fasting. D. all of the above.

| _D_ | 20. | To produce a healthy infant, the mother should ideally have an adequate diet: |

A. during the 9 months she carries the infant.
B. during the last trimester, when the baby is growing so rapidly.
C. during the second and third trimesters of pregnancy.
D. beginning long before conception occurs and continuing through the period of lactation.

| _D_ | 21. | Select the following factor that is least likely to pose a risk to maternal and fetal health during pregnancy and childbirth. |

A. underweight mother
B. maternal age 15 years or under
C. many closely spaced pregnancies
D. maternal age of 30 to 35 years

| _B_ | 22. | To avoid constipation, the pregnant woman should increase her intake of: |

A. milk and dairy products.
B. whole-grain bread, bran, and fruits.
C. sugars and starches.
D. lean meat, poultry, and fish.

| _C_ | 23. | The practice of eating dirt, clay, or laundry starch during pregnancy is called: |

A. meconium.
B. cretinism.

C. pica.
D. pregnancy-induced hypertension.

| _D_ | 24. | Advantages and benefits of breast-feeding to the mother include all but which of the following? |

A. greater convenience
B. a more rapid loss of the fat tissue that may have accumulated in her body during pregnancy
C. fosters close contact between mother and infant
D. less nutritional demands on the mother

| _B_ | 25. | Infants born after normal gestation length, but weighing less than 5-1/2 pounds are labeled: |

A. low birth weight.
B. small for gestational age.
C. premature.
D. normal, the smaller the better.

Answers to selected questions

IV. B.
a. vitamin B-6 and amino acids -- chicken meets both needs
b. calcium and vitamin D -- fortified milk meets both needs
c. thiamin and riboflavin -- enriched breads meets both needs
d. vitamin C -- oranges; amino acids -- chicken
e. iron -- beef, folate -- spinach
f. potassium and vitamin A -- apricots meets both needs

VI. birth defects; in utero

Chapter 14
Nutrition From Infancy Through Adolescence

I. **Points to consider**

Chapter 14 is designed to allow you to:

1. Describe how nutrition affects infant growth and physiological development.

2. Outline the diet guidelines to meet the basic nutritional needs for normal growth and development for the infant and discuss some do's and don'ts associated with infant feeding.

3. List several challenges parents must face in dealing with childhood eating habits.

4. List the nutrients often found to be lacking in the diet of infants, toddlers, preschoolers, and teenagers and make recommendations to remedy the problems.

5. Distinguish between food allergies and intolerances and make recommendations for treating both.

II. **Word parts**

Complete the following exercise using words in Chapter 14.

Word Part	Meaning	Examples
pharmac	related to a medicine or drug	______________
plas	to form	______________
troph	nutrition	______________
arche	beginning	______________
andr	male	______________
gen	produce	______________
cyto	cell	______________

III. **Flash cards**

Cut out and review the flash cards for this chapter in Appendix A.

IV.   Review and synthesis

A.   "From observations of Egyptian mummies we see that infants were about the same size in 300 BC as they are today. However, adult mummies are much smaller than adults are today." (443)

1.   Nutrient needs increase during the first year of life. For the following nutrients, describe one function in relation to growth and development.

	Nutrients	Function
a.	protein	_________________________
b.	vitamin A	_________________________
c.	vitamin C	_________________________
d.	vitamin D	_________________________
e.	iron	_________________________
f.	calcium	_________________________
g.	zinc	_________________________

See Chapters 7, 8, and 9 in your textbook if you need to refresh your memory.

2.   What are three potential advantages of using formula feeding to obtain these nutrients from the parents' standpoint? (448)

a.

b.

c.

B.   "A common reason offered for introducing solid foods early--before 4 to 6 months of age -- is the belief that it helps the infant sleep through the night. However, many studies have shown that sleeping through the night is a developmental milestone for the infant." (452-453)

1.   Discuss three reasons why solid foods are not recommended for an infant during the first few months of life.

a.

b.

c.

2.   Describe one approach for the introduction of semisolid foods and table foods in infancy. (453)

	Age (months)		
	4 to 6	6 to 8	9 to 12

In the boxes, put foods to start at the ages indicated.

C.   "Parents may wonder whether it is important to limit children's saturated fat and cholesterol intake to minimize risk of future heart disease." What current recommendations would you give parents concerning the use of fat, cholesterol, salt, and sugar in the diet of an infant? (456)

a.   Fat

b.   Cholesterol

c.   Salt

d.   Sugar

D.   "The rapid growth rate that characterizes infancy quickly tapers during the next few years. The average weight gain is only 5 pounds during the second year of life." A 2-year-old's mother is discussing the child's nutritional needs with you. The mother is concerned because the child is eating less than what her mother thinks the 2-year-old should be eating. She is gaining weight and growing normally, but the mother states that the child had a better appetite a year ago. Should this mother be concerned? Why or why not? (462)

E.   "Surprisingly, children eat what they are exposed to. At this age children can eat a well-rounded and healthy diet if served to them."

1.   List four general guidelines to follow when planning diets for preschoolers. (463)

a.

b.

c.

d.

2.	Outline a food plan for a 5-year-old girl, and then in the right-hand column develop a 1-day diet. (463)

Food group	Number of servings	Actual foods to help meet recommendation
Milk, yogurt, and cheese		
Meat, poultry, fish, dry beans, eggs and nuts		
Vegetables		
Fruits		
Breads, cereals, rice, and pasta		

F.   "Teenage girls especially are very concerned with weight gain, appearance, and acceptability."

1.   Adolescents pose nutritional concerns as a result of their lifestyles. List three lifestyle characteristics that may jeopardize their nutritional status. (467)

     a.

     b.

     c.

2.   List the two potential advantages and disadvantages of snacking during the teen years. (469)

<u>Advantages</u>	<u>Disadvantages</u>
a.	a.
b.	b.

V. **Applying nutrition to your life**

"Major scientific groups, such as the American Dietetic Association and the American Society for Clinical Nutrition, believe that vitamin and mineral supplements are unnecessary for healthy children. It is better to focus on good foods." (464)   Find the listing of a school lunch menu in your local newspaper, or use the following one. Using the computer software or Appendix A in your textbook, do a nutritional analysis for the following nutrients for a 9-year-old boy you are baby-sitting for a week while his parents are in Europe.

<u>Your menu</u>	<u>Sample menu</u>	<u>Approximate serving size</u>
	pepperoni pizza	4-1/2 ounces (135 grams)
	chocolate chip cookie	3/4 ounce (21 grams)
	banana	1/2 of large size
	2% low-fat milk	1 cup

	<u>Nutrient intake from meal</u>	<u>one third of RDA for 9-year-old boy</u>
Energy (kcals)	_____________	_____________
Protein (g)	_____________	_____________
Vitamin A (RE)	_____________	_____________
Thiamin (mg)	_____________	_____________
Riboflavin (mg)	_____________	_____________
Vitamin C (mg)	_____________	_____________
Calcium (mg)	_____________	_____________
Iron (mg)	_____________	_____________

VI.   **Chapter 14 summary**

Fill in the blanks using the words listed at the end of this summary.

Growth is very rapid during infancy; birth weight doubles in _______ months, and length increases by __________ in the first year. An adequate diet, especially protein intake, is very important to support normal growth. Malnutrition can cause irreversible changes in growth and development. Growth in an infant and child is monitored by measuring body weight, __________ (or length), and head circumference over time. Nutrient needs in the first 6 months can be met by __________ or formula. Supplementary __________ and iron may be needed in the first 6 months for breast-fed infants, and supplemental __________ may be needed by both breast-fed and formula-fed infants.

Infant formulas generally contain lactose or sucrose, heat-treated proteins from cow's milk, and vegetable oil. Formulas may or may not be fortified with ______. Sanitation is very important in preparing and storing formula. Solid food should not be added to an infant's diet until there is a __________, the gastrointestinal tract is able to digest these complex foods, the infant has the __________ to swallow voluntarily and control tongue thrusting, and the risk of developing ________ decreases. For most infants this readiness for solid food occurs between 4 to 6 ______ of age. The first solid food given could be iron-fortified ________, with very gradual addition of other foods, one at a time per ________. Some foods to avoid giving infants in the first year include ________, ________ cow's milk, overly salty or sweet foods, or foods that may cause choking. Introduction of iron-containing solid food at the appropriate time and avoidance of too much ________ can generally prevent ________ anemia in later infancy.

Obese children and adolescents are more likely to become obese __________ and so incur greater health risks. Parents can provide healthy food choices, while __________ should control portion sizes. When controlled early, a problem of obesity may __________ as the child continues to grow in height. Obese _________, on the other hand, do not necessarily go on to become obese children.

A slower rate of growth in the preschool years makes the choice of _____________ foods and a reduction in serving size important. Iron-rich foods, such as __________, are an important part of the Food Guide Pyramid at this age. Teens should focus on adequate iron and _____________ in the diet. This is especially important for girls as they strive to moderate high __________ food choices.

_____________ does not appear to be related to eating chocolate or any other specific foods. It is caused by overactive _____________ (sebaceous) glands that respond, in part, to high _____________ levels. Treatment options now include acutane, a _____________ derivative.

Food allergies may be caused by __________ responses to food. Elimination or a reduction in the use of allergy-causing foods can bring relief. _____________ an infant is a wise preventative step for future generations. Food _________ are not caused by allergic responses, but rather by offending substances in foods, such as lactose in the presence of low intestinal lactase levels, or <u>Salmonella</u> bacteria toxins.

Use the following words to complete the summary

acne	food allergies	iron	self-correct
adults	height	iron deficiency	testosterone
breast-feeding	honey	lean red meats	vitamin A
calcium	human milk	low-fat	vitamin D
children	immune	months	week
cow's milk	infants	nutrient-dense	4 to 6
fat	infant cereals	nutritional need	50 %
fat-secreting	intolerances	physical ability	
fluoride			

Check your answers using the summary for Chapter 14 in the textbook and the next page of this <u>Study Guide</u> for the last seven answers.

VII.   Practice examination

Cover the answers on your initial attempt.

__B__   1.   The solid food(s) usually first added to the infant's diet is (are):

    A. milk.   C. fruits.
    B. iron-fortified cereals.   D. vegetables.

__C__   2.   Which of the following nutrients are needed for the synthesis of protein tissue in both the fetus and the newborn?

    A. vitamin C, vitamin D, and niacin
    B. vitamin A, copper, and calcium
    C. vitamin B-6, vitamin B-12, and zinc
    D. thiamin, niacin, and riboflavin

__C__   3.   During the late childhood and adolescent periods, the RDA are greatly increased for:

    A. vitamin A, vitamin D, and calcium.
    B. vitamin C, folate, and zinc.
    C. calcium, phosphorus, and iron.
    D. vitamin B-6, vitamin B-12, and folate.

__A__   4.   The nutrients most often deficient in the diets of American adolescents are:

    A. calcium and iron.
    B. protein and vitamin C.
    C. thiamin and iron.
    D. calcium and vitamin D.

__B__   5.   Obese children should strive to:

    A. ignore their problem.
    B. maintain their weight and "grow into it".
    C. avoid salt.
    D. lose weight until it is desirable for height.

__D__   6.   A newborn baby should triple his or her birth weight by about _____ of age?

    A. 10 months   C. 8 months
    B. 6 months   D. 12 months

__B__   7.   The cutoff for low-birth-weight babies is _____ kilograms.

    A. 2.1   C. 2.7
    B. 2.5   D. 2.3

__D__   8.   Most health authorities recommend that solid food should be given to the infant at what age?

    A. 3 to 4 months   C. 2 months
    B. 1 month   D. 4 to 6 months

_C_   9.   When children are about 1 year of age, their appetite decreases. This is caused by:

A. dislike of foods served.
B. more interest in the environment.
C. decrease in growth rate.
D. loss of interest in food.

_A_   10.   A good rule of thumb for feeding preschool children is _____ of each food served for each year of age.

A. 1 tablespoon   C. 3 tablespoons
B. 2 tablespoons   D. 4 tablespoons

_B_   11.   Protein allowances for infants are about _____ per kilogram of body weight per day.

A. 1 gram   C. 4 grams
B. 2 grams   D. 8 grams

_D_   12.   A food allergen can be identified by:

A. the child's likes and dislikes for foods.
B. noting the symptoms; milk causes a skin rash whereas chocolate causes diarrhea.
C. noting what was eaten at the last meal.
D. a trial of food elimination and later challenge feeding of the suspected food.

_C_   13.   Nutrients that may be low in infant vegetarian diets are:

A. folate and vitamin C.
B. vitamin A and vitamin C.
C. vitamin B-12 and zinc.
D. protein and thiamin.

_C_   14.   Which of the following factors is NOT a predictor of later obesity?

A. time spent watching television
B. family history of obesity
C. number of siblings
D. weight at 6 to 8 years of age

_A_   15.   It is recommended that honey not be part of an infant's diet because it:

A. is linked to infant botulism.
B. is too high in kcalories.
C. causes constipation.
D. has low bioavailability for glucose.

_C_   16.   It is unwise to leave a bottle in the infant's mouth after he or she falls asleep because:

A. the infant will ingest too much sodium.
B. this practice may lead to obesity.
C. this practice may cause tooth decay.
D. this practice may cause tooth distortion.

_D_   17.   The WIC program is primarily for:

A. pregnant women until delivery only.
B. school age children until age 7 years.
C. school age children until age 10 years.
D. pregnant women and children up to 5 years of age.

__C__   18.   Skim milk is not recommended for children under ______ of age.

    A. 6 months   C. 2 years
    B. 1 year   D. 5 years

__A__   19.   The major problem with fast foods for adolescents is that these are:

    A. often high in fat and kcalories, and often low in calcium and fiber.
    B. too expensive for the amount of nutritive value they contribute.
    C. low in iron, thiamin, riboflavin, and niacin.
    D. too high in sugar.

__A__   20.   If a 1-year-old child wants to spoon-feed himself clumsily, the parent should:

    A. let the child try so he or she will learn.
    B. gently take the spoon away and feed him or her.
    C. use behavior modification techniques.
    D. let the child eat with his or her fingers instead.

__D__   21.   The food needs of children are so great in proportion to the size of their digestive tracts that it becomes important to:

    A. avoid liquids until after meals.
    B. serve only highly concentrated foods.
    C. provide vitamin supplements.
    D. serve snacks in addition to meals.

__C__   22.   During the first year of life, the infant increases in length by ______ over what it was at birth.

    A. 33%   C. 50%
    B. 100%   D. 20%

__D__   23.   The nutrient most often low in the diets of young children in the United States is:

    A. vitamin A.   C. vitamin C.
    B. protein.   D. iron.

__A__   24.   The food intake of preschoolers is often highly variable because:

    A. rates of growth vary.
    B. milk is often under-consumed.
    C. children are poor judges of their own appetite.
    D. children watch too much television.

__C__   25.   Symptoms of the classical allergy include all the following except:

    A. itching.   C. vomiting.
    B. reddening skin.   D. asthma.

Chapter 15
Nutrition for Adult and Elderly Years

I.   Points to consider

Chapter 15 is designed to allow you to:

1.   Discuss the cause of the principal nutrition problems of adults.

2.   List biological changes that occur during the aging process and discuss how these changes affect nutrient needs of the elderly.

3.   Identify several theories on the causes of aging.

4.   Make recommendations for dietary changes in the prevention and treatment of nutritional problems in the elderly.

5.   List several nutritional programs that are available to help meet nutritional needs of the elderly.

6.   Define Alzheimer's disease and outline its progression and relationship to nutritional status of the elderly.

7.   Characterize the effects of alcohol on the health and nutritional status of an individual.

II.   Word parts

Complete the following exercise using words in Chapter 15.

Word Part	Meaning	Examples
ger	old age	__________________
morbid	sickness	__________________
mort	death	__________________
auto	self	__________________
chron	time	__________________
ostomy	form an opening	__________________

III.   Flash cards

Cut out and review the flash cards for this chapter in Appendix A.

IV.   Review and synthesis

A.   "In general, American adults are trying to follow the diet recommendations outlined in the Dietary Guidelines." Summarize three changes adults have made to improve their diet. Then suggest some change that still should be made. (481)

<u>Positive changes</u>   <u>Needed changes</u>

a.   a.

b.   b.

c.   c.

B.   1.   "The 'graying' of America poses some problems." What are we referring to in the above quote? (485)

2.   "Life expectancy is the time an average person can expect to live." How has one's life expectancy changed in the United States over the last 80 years? (484)

3.   "One view of aging describes it as a process of slow cell death beginning soon after fertilization." Summarize how aging is related to a loss in organ reserve capacity. (485)

C.   "Although the causes of aging remain a mystery, many theories have been promoted to explain it:" Briefly describe three theories of the cause of aging. (488)

a.

b.

c.

D.	"Elderly people vary more in health status among themselves than does any other age group. This means that chronological age is not so useful in predicting physical health status." Give two examples of how each of the physiological changes below can affect nutritional status and overall health of the elderly. (489)

   a.	Decreased filtration rate by the kidneys

   b.	Decreased production of digestive enzymes and acid

   c.	Decreased motility of the digestive tract

   d.	Loss of teeth

   e.	Decreased sense of taste and smell

   f.	Reduction in muscle tissue

   g.	Reduction in sense of thirst

E.	1.	"Medications and old age often go together." List three common drug-related interactions seen in the elderly. (494)

      a.

      b.

      c.

   2.	"About 12% to 14% of elderly experience significant depression." Suggest three ways depression could affect the nutritional status in the elderly. (494)

      a.

      b.

      c.

F.	"To predict the nutritional problems of an elderly person, it is necessary to know to what extent physiological capabilities have been affected by aging." (489)

    1.	List four nutrition-related diseases that occur more often in elderly adults than in other age groups. Add a dietary recommendation to help compensate for each. (489-495)

        a.

        b.

        c.

        d.

    2.	Why is a diet with a high nutrient density recommended for the elderly? (495)

G.	"Diet plans for the elderly should focus on nutrient density, especially on the nutrients vitamin D along with sun exposure, vitamins E, B-6, B-12, C, riboflavin, and thiamin, and the minerals iron, calcium, and zinc." List five general guidelines for promoting healthful eating in later years. (498)

    a.

    b.

    c.

    d.

    e.

H.	"Nutrition programs for those age 60 and over offer congregate meal programs, which provide lunch at a central location, and home-delivered meals." The U.S. government sets specific standards for home-served meals and for those served in congregate feeding centers. List two of these meal standards. (500)

    a.

    b.

V.   **Applying nutrition to your life**

"Diet plans for the elderly should focus on nutrient density." (495) Take a look at how eating quick service food can affect adult nutrition. Using the information in Appendix A in your textbook or the computer software program, answer the following questions.

1.   If your diet allows you to eat between 500 and 650 kcalories of hamburger on a bun, which of the following would be the most nutritious choice?

    a.   McDonald's Big Mac hamburger
    b.   Burger King's Whopper sandwich

Why did you choose the one you did? On what nutrients did you base your decision?

2.   Perform an analysis of the following choices from a quick service restaurant diet for someone 30 years older than you, but of your weight, height, and gender. Compare the amounts of kcalories, vitamin A, vitamin B-6, folate, vitamin C, iron, calcium, zinc, to the RDA for elderly persons.

<u>Breakfast</u>

4 ounces orange juice
2 Egg McMuffins
2 cups black coffee

<u>Lunch</u>

1 Burger King Whopper
1 order french fries
12 ounces regular cola drink

<u>Dinner</u>

1 Arby's regular roast beef sandwich
1 order french fries
1 cup black coffee
1 Dairy Queen banana split

Which nutrients fall below 100% of the RDA?

Can you suggest simple changes to improve this diet, focusing on the nutrients showing the lowest percentages?

VI.   Chapter 15 summary

Fill in the blanks using the words listed at the end of this summary.

A goal for all of us should be to delay symptoms of and disabilities from ___________ diseases for as many years as possible. Good nutritional habits -- especially following the Food Guide Pyramid and _________________ -- play a role in this process. A basic plan for health promotion and disease prevention includes eating a proper diet, exercising regularly, abstaining from smoking, limiting alcohol intake, and limiting stress.

The 1990 Dietary Guidelines for Americans recommend that individuals eat a variety of foods; maintain a desirable __________; choose a diet low in fat, __________, and cholesterol; choose a diet rich in vegetables, fruits, and grains; use salt and __________ in moderation; and for those who drink alcoholic beverages do so in moderation. __________ background, medical conditions, and other lifestyle practices influence a person's optimal diet. While life span has not changed, life __________ has increased dramatically over the past century. For societies, this means an increasing proportion of the population is over ___________ years of age.

Aging begins before birth. Cell aging results from automatic cellular changes and ___________ influences, such as DNA damage, damage caused by electron-seeking compounds, _________ changes, high blood glucose levels, and alterations in the immune system.

Nutritional problems of the elderly are related to the presence of chronic diseases and to the normal decreases in __________ function that occur with time. These include loss of teeth, lessened sensitivity of the senses of __________ and smell, changes in gastrointestinal tract function, and deterioration in heart and __________ health. Although disease affects nutritional state, the reverse is also true. Immune function is adversely affected by __________, setting the stage for infection.

__________ disease is a progressive and irreversible brain disorder. Its causes are unknown. It differs from other types of senile dementia in that the brain tissue accumulates __________ plaques and tangled nerves. Nutritional health for people in advanced stages of this disease is often complicated by special __________ problems.

Specific nutrient requirements for the elderly are only now being studied extensively. Diet plans should be based on the Food Guide Pyramid and individualized for present health problems, decreased ___________________, the presence of drug nutrient interactions, possible depression, and economic constraints. Specific nutrients such as vitamins D, E, _____, B-6, C, and B-12, _____________, zinc, and calcium often deserve special attention in diet planning.

____________ is an issue for all adults -- from early adulthood through elderly years. Its ability to influence ___________ health is enormous. In the short run, alcohol affects the ___________ more than any other organ. Acting as a sedative, it tends to relieve the drinker's _______________, slur speech, reduce coordination in walking, and impair judgement. Drinking alcohol excessively contributes to certain forms of cancer, cirrhosis of the ____________, motor vehicle and other accidents, suicides, and homicides.

Use the following words to complete the summary

alcohol	expectancy	organ
Alzheimer's	environmental	physical abilities
anxiety	feeding	protein
body weight	genetic	saturated fat
bone	hormonal	sugar
brain	iron	taste
chronic	liver	thiamin
Dietary Guidelines	nutritional	undernutrition
		65

Check your answers using the summary for Chapter 15 in your textbook, and the next page of this <u>Study Guide</u> for the last five answers.

VI. alcohol, nutritional, brain, anxiety, liver

VII.   Practice examination

Cover the answers on your initial attempt.

_A_   1.   Experiments on animals show that the animals who lived the longest were:

A. fed nutritionally balanced diets that contained fewer kcalories than the amounts
   normally eaten by the animal.
B. fed the amounts normally eaten by the animal, but the supply of each specific
   nutrient was carefully controlled to ensure it always met the RDA.
C. fed nutritious diets in larger amounts than normally consumed by the animal.
D. allowed to eat as much as they wanted at any time they wanted.

_D_   2.   The reason the incidence of obesity increases with age is that:

A. the basal metabolic rate decreases with age.
B. physical activity often decreases with age.
C. kcalorie intake exceeds kcalorie expenditure.
D. all of the above.

_B_   3.   The deficiency of which of the following nutrients may result in anemia?

A. phosphorus, iron, protein, or selenium
B. iron, folate, vitamin B-6, or vitamin B-12
C. calcium, magnesium, folate, or iron
D. vitamin C, protein, iron, or manganese

_C_   4.   To maintain optimal nutritional status and proper weight, the diet of an elderly person must have a
           __________ nutrient density and be __________ in kcalories.

A. low, high   C. high, moderate
B. low, low   D. high, high

_C_   5.   During aging, the needs for vitamins and minerals generally:

A. continually fluctuate.   C. remain constant.
B. greatly decrease.   D. greatly increase.

_A_   6.   Theories on aging include all <u>except</u> which of the following ideas?

A. reduced physical activity spares physiological deterioration.
B. cell loss is genetically programmed.
C. partial misdirection of the immune system occurs.
D. intracellular sludge accumulates.

_A_   7.   During mid-life, the most important component of the diet to adjust is:

          A. kcalorie intake.   C. carbohydrate intake.
          B. water intake.   D. vitamin intake.

_A_   8.   Some ways to reduce the risk of coronary heart disease are:

          A. quit smoking and reduce saturated fat intake.
          B. reduce exercise to prevent stress on the heart.
          C. obtain 50% of total kcalories from fat and decrease carbohydrate intake.
          D. all of the above.

_D_   9.   Which of the following does **NOT** describe a physiological change of aging?

          A. decreases in digestion and absorption capacity
          B. reduction in lean body mass
          C. lower basal metabolism
          D. increase in taste sensitivity

_C_   10.   The two key terms for adequate adult nutrition are:

          A. varied and minimum amounts.
          B. colorful foods and abundance.
          C. varied and appropriate amounts.
          D. similar and adequate.

_A_   11.   Recommendations for preventing osteoporosis include:

          A. consuming adequate amounts of calcium from infancy throughout adulthood.
          B. consuming more potassium and selenium.
          C. increasing the intake of iron, magnesium, and zinc during adulthood.
          D. A and B.

_C_   12.   Of the following, the principal nutrition problem of young and middle-aged adults is:

          A. anemia.   C. obesity.
          B. goiter.   D. hypoglycemia.

_A_   13.   The maximum life span for humans is:

          A. 100 to 120 years.   C. 70 to 80 years.
          B. 40 to 60 years.   D. 65 years.

_C_   14.   Common nutrition-related diseases of adults include:

          A. asthma, diabetes, and hypertension.
          B. hypertension, cancer and arthritis.
          C. atherosclerosis, hypertension, and obesity.
          D. atherosclerosis, hypertension, and kidney disease.

_A_   15.   Some nutrient needs in adulthood are lowered because of decreased needs for:

          A. growth.   C. physical activity.
          B. maintenance.   D. regulation of body processes.

| B | 16. | To combat the high incidence of overweight and obesity in the United States, many people are reducing their intake of: |

A. whole-grain cereals.   C. cholesterol.
B. total kcalories.   D. sodium.

| A | 17. | Americans have reduced intakes of cholesterol and saturated fat in the past few years to decrease the risk of: |

A. coronary heart disease.   C. anemia.
B. colon cancer.   D. osteoporosis.

| D | 18. | Because of the high incidence of hypertension in the United States, many people are encouraged to lower their intake of: |

A. meats.   C. dairy products.
B. sugars and sweets.   D. sodium.

| C | 19. | To help prevent colon cancer, Americans today are increasing their intake of: |

A. fresh fruit.   C. whole-grain cereals.
B. lean, red meat.   D. dairy fats.

| B | 20. | During adulthood, the component of the diet that most often needs reexamination is: |

A. water.   C. carbohydrate.
B. energy.   D. vitamin.

| D | 21. | At the turn of the century the most common cause of death was: |

A. cancer.   C. accidents.
B. heart disease.   D. infectious diseases.

| D | 22. | Nutrition programs such as congregate meals or home-delivered meals provide which of the following? |

A. an improved nutritional status
B. a social atmosphere
C. an economical meal for low income elderly
D. all of the above

| B | 23. | Drinking out of aluminum cans causes Alzheimer's Disease. |

A. True   B. False

| D | 24. | Among the older population of the United States, the fastest growing segment of the population is ages: |

A. 60 to 65   C. 70 to 80
B. 65 to 70   D. 85 +

| D | 25. | The fluid recommendation for the elderly is the same as for younger adults, |

A. about 1 milliliter per kcalorie of energy metabolized.
B. about 2 liters a day.
C. about 8 cups of fluid daily
D. either a, b, or c.

Chapter 16
Taking Charge of Your Diet

I. **Points to consider**

Chapter 16 is designed to allow you to:

1. Outline the behavior change process.

2. Describe how to set goals and develop contracts to help meet these goals.

3. List how to modify habits and environments to encourage desired behavior changes.

4. State techniques to prevent behavior change relapse.

5. List some techniques for dining defensively.

6. Compare and contrast various traditional foods in several ethnic diets.

7. Evaluate the pros and cons of "eating on the run."

II. **Word parts**

Complete the following exercise using words in Chapter 16.

Word Part	Meaning	Examples
arthr	joint	_______________
psych	organ of thought and reason	_______________
gno	to know	_______________
lapse	to slip or fall back	_______________

III. **Flash cards**

Cut out and review the flash cards for this chapter in Appendix A.

IV. **Review and synthesis**

A. "Behavior patterns that have evolved throughout a lifetime do not change or disappear overnight. Planned behavior changes occur gradually and with some effort." Briefly describe five steps in behavior change. (516)

a.

b.

c.

d.

e.

B. "Having decided to attempt a change, the person begins a trial run." Outline the benefits and costs for changing one of your "problem" food behaviors. (517)

Benefits of changing the behavior.	Costs of changing the behavior.
Benefits of not changing the behavior.	Costs of not changing the behavior.

C. "Whatever is pushing you to deviate from your plan, substitute another behavior for it." Identify the links that make up one of your "problem" behaviors on the following diagram. Draw a line through the chain where it might be interrupted. Then add a link at that spot to fasten the beginning of a better outcome to the initial stimulus. Briefly describe the new desired outcome. (531)

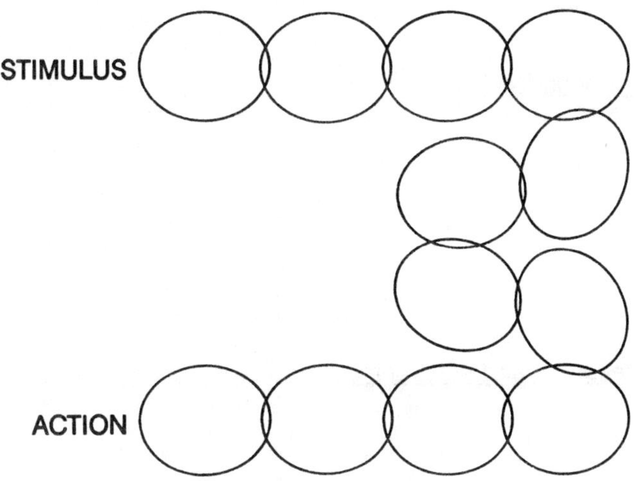

D. "Recruit support from others -- have some family members, roommates, or friends witness your contract, educate them about the program and your needs." Outline four tips that could help you prepare to change a problem food behavior. (526)

a.

b.

c.

d.

E. "Relapse often starts with a high-risk situation. Most people at first don't recognize the conditions that promote the relapse. One 'slip' sometimes snowballs into a series of lapses that lead to complete reversion into old behaviors." How do you think relapse into previous food habits is best minimized? Describe four methods. (528)

a.

b.

c.

d.

V.   Applying nutrition to your life

"Many things can trigger inappropriate eating behavior. But effective tactics can be used to gain control of eating." List some tactics you could use for managing your "problem" food behaviors in the following situations. (522)

<u>Buying and storing food</u>

a.

b.

<u>Cooking, preparing, and serving food</u>

a.

b.

<u>Eating food</u>

a.

b.

<u>Eating in restaurants</u>

a.

b.

<u>Coping with emotions, as well as other people</u>

a.

b.

Fill in the blanks using the words listed at the end of this summary.

Behavior change occurs in a progression of steps. First, persons become ______ of a problem. Then they open themselves to new information about it, evolving a ____________. They undertake a _______ for the change, during which time positive reinforcement is critical. If an initial trial is successful, persons may permanently ________ new behaviors. Before charting a behavior plan, it is important to discover personal _________ regarding the behavior. A _______ can be kept for a week or more. This may show eating patterns and other behaviors that either contribute to or discourage new behaviors. This exercise also helps reveal areas of the external environment that need to be altered to reduce temptation.

When setting goals for a behavior plan, it is best to focus on _________ that lead to an intended result. Building ________ reinforcement into the plan to reward achievements helps maintain momentum. After setting a plan of action, it is often helpful to develop a _______ that lists the actions intended to occur, the positive _________ to be received, and the _______ for the behavior change. The __________ should at first reward positive ______ and later reward ultimate objectives. Before embarking on a behavior change program, the person should evaluate personal _______. A plan, no matter how skillfully developed, will not succeed unless a person has a strong desire to achieve the ________.

To implement a plan, it is important to monitor ________ and provide _______. Controlling one's ________ can reduce temptations to deviate from the plan. Small ______ should be expected and not be seen as an excuse to abandon change. A ________ attitude can prevent collapse of the whole strategy. The person should ________ into a plan for the possibility of ________. Most people revert to previous behaviors at times, especially during periods of stress or interpersonal conflict.

Choosing ___________ foods is not so difficult in many of today's quick service restaurants. Some restaurants have evolved beyond hamburgers, French fries and milk shakes to include a variety of vegetables, ___________, and ethnic foods. Still, of the kcalories in most quick service choices about ___ come from ___________. Thus, many of these meal selections are high kcalorie options when compared to the amount of other nutrients provided. A close look at fat intake and use of the ___________ aids in making wise food choices.

Use the following words to complete the summary

adopt	food diary	reward
aware	goals	salad bars
balanced	Food Guide Pyramid	small steps
behaviors	healthy	supplements
commitment	positive	strengths and weaknesses
contract	progress	time frame
environment	receptive framework	trial period
failures	reinforcement	40% to 50%
fat	relapse	
forgive-and forget		

Check your answers using the summary for Chapter 16 in your textbook and page 188 of this <u>Study Guide</u> for the last five answers.

VIII.   Practice examination

Cover the answers on your initial attempt.

__B__   1.   Behavior change:

A. is mostly a matter of willpower.
B. depends on a well-considered plan.
C. usually happens spontaneously.
D. requires the help of a professional.

__D__   2.   Which of the following should be included in a food diary?

A. time of day   C. mood
B. foods eaten and amount   D. all of the above

__A__   3.   The best way to make a behavior change is to:

A. attempt a series of small changes leading to the goal.
B. address the entire problem at once.
C. wait until your current behavior is dangerous.
D. set lofty goals.

__D__   4.   The first step in the behavior change process is:

A. self-criticism.   C. trial change.
B. adaptation.   D. awareness.

__C__   5.   Success at changing a behavior depends on:

A. the nature of the problem.   C. commitment.
B. willpower.   D. strategy.

__B__   6.   Actual food choices are primarily determined by:

A. cost.   C. health value.
B. sensory appeal.   D. convenience.

__D__   7.   A good plan for behavior change should:

A. focus on specific, measurable goals.
B. include appropriate rewards along the way.
C. allow for revision as needed.
D. all of the above.

__C__   8.   Distorting information and denying facts to support wishful thinking is defined as:

A. behavior chains.   C. rationalization.
B. contingency management.   D. positive reinforcement.

__D__   9.   If a lapse occurs:

A. realize that you are only human and plan to prevent other lapses.
B. it is an indication that your plan is unsuccessful.
C. it may be an indication of stress or internal conflict.
D. A and C

_D_   10.   Eating patterns are difficult to change because:

A. eating is closely tied to social occasions.
B. people eat not only for hunger, but pleasure.
C. people may use food to fight boredom, stress, or loneliness.
D. all of the above.

_D_   11.   Which one of the following cooking techniques does not promote less fat?

A. broiling. C. roasting.
B. stir-frying. D. breading.

_B_   12.   Quick service foods are often high in __________, and so choices should be made carefully.

A. carbohydrate C. protein
B. fat D. dietary fiber

_D_   13.   Behavior modification is defined as:

A. recognizing which foods are high in kcalories.
B. accepting the fact that people are fat because of a genetic predisposition.
C. accepting psychological counseling for eating problems.
D. finding ways to modify behaviors that contribute to health problems.

_A_   14.   Forming a plan of action to respond to environmental conditions when overeating is likely is designated by weight-loss professionals as:

A. contingency management.
B. self-monitoring.
C. stimulus control.
D. restraint.

Answers to selected questions

VI. healthy; salad bars; 40% to 50%; fat; Food Guide Pyramid

Chapter 17
Food Safety

I. Points to consider

Chapter 17 is designed to allow you to:

1. List some of the types of microorganisms, viruses, and parasites found in food and their general characteristics.

2. Describe the procedures that can be used to control microbial growth in foods.

3. Outline the major types of food-borne illness caused by microorganisms.

4. Compare and contrast food preservation methods and how they may contribute to the risk of food-borne illness.

5. Describe the main reasons for using chemical additives in foods, the general classes of additives, and the functions of each class.

6. List the major categories of common food additives and foods in which they are used.

7. Differentiate between food additives as intentional or unintentional, and describe the importance of the Generally Recognized As Safe (GRAS) list and the Delaney clause.

II. Word parts

Complete the following exercise using words in Chapter 17.

Word Part	Meaning	Examples
ferment	leaven	__________________
cocci	berry shape	__________________
septic	due to decomposition	__________________
micro	small	__________________
sequester	separate from the whole	__________________
botul(us)	sausage	__________________

III. Flash cards

Cut out and review the flash cards for this chapter in Appendix A.

IV.   Review and synthesis

A.   "Today, we know that cleanliness, keeping hot foods hot and cold foods cold, and cooking foods thoroughly offer additional protection from food-borne illness."

1.   List 4 factors that are responsible for food spoilage. (544)

   a.

   b.

   c.

   d.

2.   Using the thermometer, indicate: (546)

Degrees Celsius (° C)		Degrees Fahrenheit (° F)
100		212
74		165
60		140
5		40
0		32
-18		0

   a.   refrigerator temperature

   b.   danger zone: where bacteria grow

   c.   minimum temperature to cook beef

   d.   minimum temperature to cook pork

   e.   ideal temperature range for microbes that cause food-borne illness

B.   "Because each teaspoon of soil contains about 2 billion bacteria, we are constantly at risk for food-borne illness. Luckily, only a small number of these bacteria actually pose a threat." (541)

1.   What is the cause of most food-borne illness?

2.   What are some other possible causes of food-borne illness?

    a.

    b.

    c.

3.   List six general guidelines to follow to avoid food-borne illness. (546)

    a.

    b.

    c.

    d.

    e.

    f.

4. For the following organisms and agents that cause food-borne illness, list their source, symptoms, and specific prevention measures. (542)

	Source	Symptoms	Specific prevention measures
<u>Staphylococcus aureus</u>			
<u>Salmonella</u>			
<u>Clostridium perfringens</u>			
<u>Clostridium botulinum</u>			

C. 1. "In 1958, all food additives used in the United States and considered safe at that time were put on a <u>Generally Recognized As Safe (GRAS)</u> list." Briefly define the GRAS list in terms of its development and use. (552)

2. "If an additive is shown to cause cancer, even though caused by very high doses, no margin of safety is allowed. The food additive <u>cannot</u> be used because it would violate the <u>Delaney clause</u> in the 1958 Food Additive Amendments." What arguments could you use to support and to refute the use of the Delaney clause? (553)

<u>For</u>

<u>Against</u>

D.   "Limiting food spoilage accounts for the bulk of food additive use." (556)

1.   Additives are used in food processing for four major purposes. Match each type of additive below to the major purpose.

<u>Additive</u>   <u>Purpose</u>

a. _______   antioxidants   A. increase nutritive value

b. _______   colors   B. preserve freshness

c. _______   emulsifiers   C. aid in processing

d. _______   thiamin and   D. improve flavor or appearance
             riboflavin

e. _______   flavor enhancers

f. _______   antimicrobial agents

g. _______   stabilizers,
             thickeners, texturizers

2.   Match some common examples of additives to one of the purposes above.

a. _____ nitrates/nitrites   e. _____ monosodium glutamate (MSG)

b. _____ calcium propionate   f. _____ BHA/BHT

c. _____ potassium iodide   g. _____ sulfur dioxide

d. _____ calcium   h. _____ monoglycerides, diglycerides

See pages 198 of this <u>Study Guide</u> to check your answers to Part 1 and Part 2.

E.   "The question shouldn't be whether a food additive such as salt is a chemical, but rather is the chemical additive safe to use." (559) Using Appendix N in your textbook as needed, decipher the role of each ingredient in this food label.

INGREDIENTS: ENRICHED FLOUR, (BLEACHED WHEAT FLOUR, NIACIN, IRON, THIAMIN MONONITRATE, AND RIBOFLAVIN), VEGETABLE SHORTENING (CONTAINS ONE OR BOTH OF THE FOLLOWING PARTIALLY HYDROGENATED OILS: SOYBEAN, COTTONSEED), SODIUM ALUMINUM PHOSPHATE, MONOCALCIUM PHOSPHATE MONO- AND DIGLYCERIDES, WHEY, SALT, DRIED BUTTERMILK.

Does it make you feel more comfortable to understand <u>what actually</u> is in your food?

F.   "Farmers know potatoes must be stored in the dark so that solanine will not be synthesized." Name two natural toxicants that occur in foods and briefly describe their toxic effects. (560)

a.

b.

G.   List five environmental contaminants in food and where they are most likely to be found. (560)

a.

b.

c.

d.

e.

H.   "Ice crystals in frozen foods are not heated well by the microwave oven." Name 3 practices that can reduce the risk of bacteria surviving during microwave cooking. (547)

      a.

      b.

      c.

V.   **Applying nutrition to your life**

"Microbes that cause food-borne illness typically enter food through cross-contamination (usually from improper food handling) and grow because they are maintained at temperatures favorable to them." Assess the potential for food-borne illness where you live. Can you find poor practices in: (545)

      a.   grocery-shopping habits

      b.   length of refrigerator storage

      c.   improper cleaning of the kitchen cutting board after contact with raw meats

      d.   extent of cooking

      e.   attention to leftovers

VI.   **Chapter 17 summary**

Fill in the blanks using the words listed at the end of this summary.

___________ and other microbes in foods are the agents most likely to cause food-borne illness. To

guard against food-borne illness, in the past _______, sugar, _______, fermentation, and drying were most often used. Today, careful cooking, _______, and keeping _______ foods hot and _______ foods cold provide additional insurance. ____________ is a new, somewhat controversial, but effective "anti-spoilage" method for some foods. ___________ is a common cause of food-borne illness. It occurs when bacteria on raw animal products come in contact with foods that can support bacterial growth. Because of this risk, no food should be kept at _______ for more than _________ hours if a possibility exists that it has come in contact with raw animal products and can support bacterial growth.

Treatment for food-borne illness usually requires ___________ extra ___________, avoiding food handling while diarrhea is present, thorough _______, and bed rest. The major causes of food-borne illness today are the bacteria <u>Salmonella</u>, ____________, and ____________. To protect against the microbes, cover _______, do not sneeze on foods, avoid contact between __________ and other food products, and rapidly _______ and later thoroughly _______ leftovers. Thorough _________ and the use of ________ dairy products further protects against other bacteria and __________.

Food additives are primarily used to extend shelf life by preventing microbial growth and destruction of food components by _______, certain chemical ions, and other substances. Food additives are classified as those _________ added to foods and those that _________ end up in foods. Use of a food additive generally is limited to _______ of the greatest amount that causes no observable symptoms in animals. In most cases the _______ bans use of any intentional food additive if it causes cancer. Antioxidants, such as _______ and sulfites, prevent oxygen and enzyme destruction of food products. _________ suspend fat in ____________, improving the uniformity, smoothness, and body of foods such as ice cream. Common antimicrobial agents include ________ and sorbic acid, which prevent bacterial ______. ____________ bind free chemical ions, preventing them from causing fats to become rancid. Toxic substances occur naturally in a variety of foods, such as green potatoes, _________, and ________. Cooking foods limits their toxic effects. Environmental contaminants also can be found in food. Because most of them are _______, trim fat from meats and discard fat that is rendered during the cooking of meats, fish, and poultry. In addition, _______ fruits and vegetables thoroughly.

Most concern about pesticide residues in foods focuses on ___________ rather than acute toxicity, since the amounts of residues are extremely ___________. Growing evidence, including the problems of contamination of underground ______________, indicates that we would be better off if we ___________ our use of pesticides. Pesticide use in general substantially contributes to the ______________ applied intentionally to the earth's surface. Once a pesticide Is applied, it can turn up in a number of ___________ places. The primary reason for using pesticides is _________________.

Use the following words to complete the summary

bacteria	food irradiation	salt
chemical load	growth	sequestrants
chronic	hand washing	small
<u>Clostridium perfringens</u>	hot	smoke
cold	incidentally	sodium benzoate
cooking of foods	intentionally	<u>Staphylococcus aureus</u>
cool	moldy grains	two
cross-contamination	oxygen	unintended
cuts on hands	pasteurization	viruses
Delaney clause	pasteurized	vitamin E
drinking	raw fish	wash
economic	raw poultry products	water
emulsifiers	reduced	water supplies
fat-soluble	reheat	1/100 to 1/1000
fluids	room temperature	

Check your answers using the summary for Chapter 17 in your textbook and the next page of this <u>Study Guide</u> for the last seven answers.

IV.   D.   1. b, d, c, a, d, b, c

           2. b, b, a, a, d, b, d, c

VI.   chronic, small, water supplies, reduced, chemical load, unintended, economic

VII.   **Practice examination**

Cover the answers on your initial attempt.

__D__   1.   Food additives may be used to:

A. destroy nutrients.   C. deceive customers.
B. disguise faulty products.   D. enhance appearance.

__B__   2.   Food additives widely used for many years without apparent ill effects are on the _______ list.

A. FDA   C. additive safety
B. GRAS   D. Delaney

__A__   3.   Vitamin C, vitamin E, and BHA are all:

A. antioxidants.   C. antimicrobial agents.
B. flavor enhancers.   D. incidental food additives.

__D__   4.   It is unwise to thaw meats or poultry:

A. in a microwave oven.   C. under cool running water.
B. in the refrigerator.   D. at room temperature.

__A__   5.   Salmonella bacteria are usually spread via:

A. raw meats, poultry, and eggs.
B. pickled vegetables.
C. home-canned vegetables.
D. raw vegetables.

__A__   6.   Pasteurization involves the:

A. exposure of food to high temperatures for short periods to destroy harmful microorganisms.
B. exposure of food to heat to inactivate enzymes that cause undesirable effects in foods
   during storage.
C. the fortification of foods with vitamins A and D.
D. use of irradiation to destroy certain pathogens in foods.

__B__   7.   Which of the following is <u>NOT</u> a function of food additives?

A. emulsification
B. helps speed the cooking process
C. preservation
D. enhancement of flavor

_A_   8.   The most common cause of food-borne illness is the presence of what in foods?

        A. bacteria   C. viruses
        B. chemical preservatives   D. molds

_C_   9.   The Delaney clause states:

        A. there is a threshold for carcinogens.
        B. the Generally Recognized As Safe (GRAS) list must be reviewed every 5 years.
        C. no substance either introduced or reevaluated after 1958 that is shown to be carcinogenic can
            be knowingly added to food.
        D. additives must be evaluated for safety.

_A_   10.   The factor that is least important to control in order to limit food-borne illness is:

        A. ptomaine synthesis.   C. temperature of food.
        B. presence of microbes.   D. time of incubation.

_D_   11.   Indirect additives include:

        A. oils and fats in the forms of shortenings.
        B. substances that provide a major energy contribution to the food, such as sugar.
        C. substances often used at home, such as vanilla and garlic.
        D. minerals from cooking vessels.

_D_   12.   Ancient methods of food preservation include:

        A. pasteurizing and sterilizing.
        B. canning, blanching, and irradiating.
        C. freezing and boiling.
        D. drying, smoking, and fermenting.

_C_   13.   Regulation of food additives is the responsibility of the:

        A. American Medical Association.
        B. Department of Agriculture.
        C. Food and Drug Administration.
        D. National Research Council.

_A_   14.   Aflatoxins:

        A. are linked to cancer in animals.
        B. are intentional food additives.
        C. occur only in corn and peanut products.
        D. are on the GRAS list.

_B_   15.   Solanine is:

        A. not known to be harmful to humans.
        B. a naturally occurring toxin found in green potatoes.
        C. a naturally occurring toxin found in shellfish.
        D. a toxin that grows on corn and peanut products.

_A_   16.   Substances used to preserve foods by lowering the pH are:

        A. vinegar and citric acid.   C. baking powder and soda.
        B. smoke and irradiation.   D. salt and sugar.

_D_   17.   In foods, additives known as anticaking agents:

A. incorporate fat into water-based mediums.
B. speed up the process of aging in flour.
C. serve as a flavor enhancers.
D. absorb moisture to keep a product free-flowing.

_B_   18.   Food can be kept for long periods of time by adding salt or sugar because these substances:

A. make the food too acidic for spoilage to occur.
B. bind to water, thereby making it unavailable to the microorganisms.
C. kill microorganisms.
D. dissolve the cell walls in plant foods.

_B_   19.   A danger of using home-canned food if the processing has been inadequate is:

A. cancer.   C. excessive nutrient loss.
B. botulism.   D. excessive tin in the juice.

_D_   20.   Which of the following does not contribute to harmful bacterial growth in foods?

A. exposure to raw poultry or meat juices
·B. soil contamination in foods
C. temperatures between 40° F and 140° F
D. cooling foods to adequately low temperatures within two hours

_A_   21.   Nitrite prevents the growth of:

A. <u>C. botulinum</u>.   C. <u>S. aureus</u>.
B. <u>C. perfringens</u>.   D. yeasts.

_B_   22.   The organism that causes food-borne illness and often associated with small cuts and boils is:

A. <u>Aspergillus</u>.   C. <u>C. botulinum</u>.
B. <u>Staphylococcus</u>.   D. <u>Salmonella</u>.

_A_   23.   Bacteria that can grow in the absence of oxygen are called:

A. anaerobes.   C. aerobes.
B. molds.   D. yeasts.

_D_   24.   The organisms used in the process of fermentation:

A. metabolize all the oxygen in food.
B. produce water in the food.
C. utilize all the nutrients in a food.
D. produce products, such as acids, that inhibit the growth of other organisms.

_D_   25.   Keeping food above 140° F (60° C):

A. increases microbial growth.
B. slows chemical deterioration.
C. decreases chemical reactions.
D. reduces the growth of pathogens.

CHAPTER 18
Undernutrition Throughout the World

I. **Points to consider**

Chapter 18 is designed to allow you to:

1. Define and characterize the terms hunger, malnutrition, and undernutrition.

2. Evaluate the consequences of undernutrition during critical periods in a person's life.

3. Examine undernutrition in America and highlight several programs established to combat this problem.

4. Examine undernutrition in the Third World and evaluate the major obstacles which hinder a solution.

5. Outline some possible solutions to undernutrition in the Third World.

6. Consider how biotechnology and low input sustainable agriculture (LISA) may help solve the food shortage problem, while at the same time protect the environment.

II. **Word parts**

Complete the following exercise using words in Chapter 18.

Word Part	Meaning	Examples
mal	abnormal	__________________
gen	to become or produce	__________________
chron	pertaining to time	__________________
bio	pertaining to life	__________________
under	beneath	__________________
geo	pertaining to earth	__________________
pestis	plague	__________________
sanita	pertaining to health	__________________

III. **Flash cards**

Cut out and review the flash cards for this chapter in Appendix A.

A.   1.   "Symptoms of chronic hunger can be found not only in the developing world, but also in many people living at or below the poverty level in America and elsewhere." List four causes of chronic hunger in the United States. (573)

Causes of chronic hunger:

a.

b.

c.

d.

2.   What action would contribute to a solution for one of the four causes you listed above?

3.   "Undernutrition is the most common form of malnutrition among the poor in both developing and developed countries." Define and distinguish between the terms malnutrition, undernutrition, and protein-energy malnutrition. (573)

B.   1.   "The human organism is particularly susceptible to the effects of undernutrition during periods of rapid growth, especially during pregnancy, infancy, and childhood." Give one example of how undernutrition can jeopardize the health of a pregnant woman, an infant, and a child. (573)

<u>pregnant woman:</u>

<u>infant:</u>

<u>child:</u>

2.	List two possible reasons that the infant mortality for African Americans is higher than that for U.S. Caucasians. (582)

a.

b.

C.	1.	"In the 1950s it was assumed that all Americans had enough to eat. Nevertheless, occasional reports of undernutrition surfaced, mostly among the chronic poor." In the 1960s, several programs were started in order to reduce malnutrition. Match the following characteristics with the appropriate program. (You can use a number more than once.) (579)

Food Stamp Program	School Lunch and Breakfast Program	Women, Infants, and Children (WIC) Program
__________	__________	__________
__________	__________	__________

1.	Was revitalized by President John F. Kennedy.

2.	Is credited for the recent widespread drop in iron-deficiency anemia.

3.	Became nationally available in 1975.

4.	Provides food vouchers and nutrition education to low-income pregnant and lactating women and their young children.

5.	Stamps are used to purchase food.

6.	Enables low-income grade school students to receive meals at reduced or no cost.

D.   1.   "Programs which have proven immensely helpful in the United States would only be a starting point in the Third World." List four major obstacles Third World countries must face when dealing with undernutrition. Describe each in one sentence. (583)

         a.

         b.

         c.

         d.

    2.   Discuss how war and civil unrest specifically contribute to undernutrition. (593)

E.   1.   "For the most part, the problem is one of helping people produce much of their own needs and directing them to employment opportunities." Discuss one of these two solutions for Third World undernutrition and indicate why you feel the solution would work. (596)

    2.   How might biotechnology help reduce Third World undernutrition? (604)

V.   **Applying nutrition to your life**

Figure 18-7 shows that Ziggy is distressed over the lack of change in current world problems. (591) This chapter has likely made you aware of several problems related to undernutrition in the United States and developing countries. This week, make some contribution to society in order to help solve the problem of undernutrition. In other words, make some attempt to make a difference. Describe your activity below and then act on it. (HINT: Donation of money or volunteering at a soup kitchen are two possible options.)

VI.   **Chapter 18 summary**

Fill in the blanks using the words listed at the end of this summary.

________ is a common thread wherever people show undernutrition. Malnutrition can occur when the food supply is either ______ or abundant. The resulting deficiency conditions or degenerative diseases are influenced by _______ makeup.

Undernutrition is the most common form of _________ in developing countries. It results from inadequate intake, _______, or use of nutrients or kcalories. Many deficiency conditions then appear and infectious diseases thrive because the _______ system cannot function properly.

The greatest risk of undernutrition occurs during critical periods of _______ and development: pregnancy, infancy, and _______. Low birth weight is a leading cause of infant _________ worldwide. Many developmental problems are caused by nutritional deprivation during critical periods of _______ growth.

Undernutrition diminishes both ______ and mental capabilities. In poor countries, this is worsened by recurrent infections, poor _______ conditions, extreme weather, inadequate shelter, and exposure to _______.

In the United States, _____________ has been nonexistent since the 1930s, but undernutrition is present. Soup kitchens, food stamps, __________________, and the Supplemental Feeding Program for Women, Infants, and Children (WIC) have focused on improving the nutritional health of poor and at-risk people. These programs have proven effective in reducing ___________ when adequately funded.

Multiple factors contribute to the problem of undernutrition in Third World countries. In densely populated countries, food ________ may be inadequate and the means for distributing food may be poor. Farming methods often encourage ________, which deprives the soil of valuable nutrients, thus defeating future efforts to grow food. Poor _________ availability hampers food production. Naturally occurring devastation from droughts, excessive rainfall, _______, crop infestation, and from human causes such as urbanization, civil unrest, _________, debt, and poor sanitation all contribute to the major problem of undernutrition.

Any proposed solutions to the problem of world undernutrition must consider the interaction of ________ factors, many of which are thoroughly embedded in ________ traditions. Family planning efforts, for example, may not succeed until life ________ can be raised. Through _______, efforts should be made to improve farming methods, encourage breast-feeding, and improve sanitation and ________. Direct food aid is only a short-term solution. In what may appear to be a step backward, a focus on subsistence-level farming, away from the specialization of _________, is needed in order to increase the economic status of people reliant on traditional __________ agriculture. This is one way to gain meaningful employment and purchasing power for vast numbers of the _________ poor.

"New biotechnology," also known as __________, directly changes some of the genetic material (DNA) of organisms to improve characteristics. It uses a wide range of cell and sub-cell techniques for ________ and then placing genetic material in organisms. It allows access to a wider _________, and it permits faster and more accurate production of new and more useful microbial, ______, and animal species.

__________________________ seeks to reduce use of purchased inputs while maintaining or increasing yields and farm profits. The overall objective is to reduce _______, environmental and health _________, and natural resource degradation.

Use the following words to complete the summary

absorption	fire	plant
brain	gene pool	poverty
cash crops	genetic	rain-fed
childhood	genetic engineering	resources
cost	growth	rural
cultural	hazards	sanitary
deaths	hygiene	scarce
diseases	immune	school lunch and breakfast program
education	low input sustainable	synthesizing
erosion	agriculture	undernutrition
expectancy	malnutrition	war
famine	multiple	water
	physical	

Check your answers using the summary for Chapter 18 in your textbook and the next page of this <u>Study Guide</u> for the last seven answers.

VI.   genetic engineering, synthesizing, gene pool, plant, low input sustainable agriculture, cost, hazards

---

VII.   Practice examination

Cover the answers on your initial attempt.

__C__   1.   The largest increase in numbers of chronically hungry people currently occur in:

    A. India.   C. Africa.
    B. The United States.   D. Asia.

__B__   2.   There are an estimated _________ chronically undernourished people in the world.

    A. 75 million   C. 2.5 billion
    B. 1 billion   D. 7.3 million

__A__   3.   The primary cause of chronic hunger is:

    A. poverty.   C. inability to eat.
    B. lack of resources.   D. drought.

__D__   4.   The human organism is particularly susceptible to the effects of undernutrition during:

    A. pregnancy.   C. childhood.
    B. infancy.   D. all of the above.

__C__   5.   Primarily, the consequence of undernutrition both in the United States and worldwide can be seen through a(n):

    A. overall decrease in food consumption.
    B. decrease in the number of obese people.
    C. increase in infant mortality rate.
    D. increase in elderly mortality rate.

__C__   6.   Currently there is estimated to be approximately _________ people in the United States living at or near the poverty level.

    A. 50 million   C. 36 million
    B. 20 billion   D. 100 thousand

__B__   7.   What program has shown to be cost effective in reducing the number of premature, low-birth-weight babies?

    A. the Food Stamp Program
    B. the WIC Program
    C. the School Lunch Program
    D. the Congregate Meal Program

__C__   8.   Those at or below the poverty level spend the majority of their money on:

    A. insurance.   C. rent.
    B. food.   D. alcohol and cigarettes.

| B | 9. | Life expectancy in the United States is approximately _________ times that in Third World countries. |

A. 1.2   C. 1.75
B. 1.5   D. 2

| B | 10. | In sub-saharan Africa, a woman who is childless is often considered to be: |

A. pure.   C. poor.
B. evil.   D. elite.

| D | 11. | In India, bananas may not be fed to children because they supposedly cause: |

A. food poisoning.   C. nutrient deficiencies.
B. inhibition of growth.   D. convulsions.

| B | 12. | Which of the following would be considered a delicacy in other countries, but would be shunned in the United States? |

A. oysters   C. brown-shelled eggs
B. insects   D. pork

| D | 13. | Many of the 15 million child deaths each year in developing countries could be prevented if: |

A. technology was improved.
B. doctors were more specialized.
C. mothers would learn more about nutrition.
D. sanitation and hygiene were improved.

| A | 14. | In Third World countries, there is a growing population shift from: |

A. rural to urban centers.
B. urban to rural centers.

| C | 15. | Women in Third World countries consider the use of infant formulas as being: |

A. expensive.   C. sophisticated.
B. cost-effective.   D. wasteful.

| D | 16. | Breast milk is noted for being: |

A. hygienic.   C. nutritionally sound.
B. readily available.   D. all of the above.

| A | 17. | The World Health Organization (WHO) estimates that 1.2 billion people are without: |

A. a safe and adequate water supply.
B. home and shelter.
C. food.
D. education.

| D | 18. | Developing countries now have two thirds of the world's 8 to 12 million people with: |

A. cancer.   C. heart disease.
B. hepatitis.   D. HIV infections (AIDS).

_A_   19.   The country that carries the largest national debt is:

A. United States.
B. Brazil.
C. South Africa.
D. Mexico.

_B_   20.   What hormone produced by cattle has been known to increase milk production when injected into dairy cattle?

A. epinephrine
B. bovine somatotropin (BST)
C. estrogen
D. ADH

_D_   21.   The extreme form of chronic hunger recently seen in Ethiopia and Sudan is known as:

A. starvation.
B. malnutrition.
C. undernutrition.
D. famine.

_C_   22.   A barrier to solving undernutrition in the Third World is **NOT**:

A. external debt.
B. poor infrastructure.
C. a lack of manpower.
D. expanding population.

_B_   23.   A nutrient closely tied to immune function is:

A. calcium.
B. zinc.
C. magnesium.
D. glucose.

_C_   24.   The nutrient most associated with anemia worldwide is:

A. vitamin B-12.
B. copper.
C. iron.
D. vitamin C.

_B_   25.   The U.S. president credited with revitalization of the effort to combat hunger in America is:

A. Eisenhower.
B. Kennedy.
C. Nixon.
D. Reagan.

CHAPTER 1

Relate the terms risk factor and chronic disease.

Relate the terms hypertension, heart disease, and stroke.

Define the term diabetes.

Define the term cancer.

Define the term cirrhosis of the liver.

Define the term nutrient.

Define the term metabolism.

What do carbohydrates and glucose have in common?

Hypertension means high blood pressure. This can injure the arteries that supply blood to the heart and brain. If the injury eventually leads to death of heart tissue, that is part of what is called heart disease. If poor blood flow leads to death of brain tissue, that is referred to as a stroke.

Risk factors are characteristics that make a disease more likely to occur, such as a high blood cholesterol level making heart disease more likely to occur. By definition, a chronic disease takes a long time to develop -- chronic means "continuing for a long time."

Cancer refers to the excessive growth of one or more cells in the body, such that they do not respond to normal, physiological controls.

In diabetes insufficient amounts of insulin are produced so that blood glucose levels do not remain within normal limits. Two forms exist: insulin-dependent, which usually develops in childhood, and noninsulin-dependent, which usually develops in adulthood and is related to excess body fat.

A nutrient is a substance found in food that a human requires in the diet to maintain health.

Cirrhosis refers to substitution of the normal healthy liver cells with connective tissues, usually because a long-standing alcohol intake poisons the liver cells.

All carbohydrates are compounds formed from a mixture of carbon, hydrogen, oxygen, and other atoms. Glucose is one example of a carbohydrate.

Metabolism refers to the chemical reactions in the body. These enable cells to release energy from foods, convert one substance to another, and prepare end products for excretion.

Contrast lipids versus fats and oils.

Contrast amino acid versus protein.

What are vitamins?

Define the term mineral.

Contrast inorganic versus organic.

Define the term kcalorie.

Define the term dietary fiber.

Define the term nutritional status.

Amino acids are the building blocks of protein. Proteins generally are composed of hundreds to thousands of amino acids linked together.

Lipids include compounds that dissolve in ether or benzene. Fats and oils are two such examples. Fats are solid at room temperature, oils are liquid at room temperature; both are classed as lipids.

Minerals are atoms (elements) that both form integral parts of the body structure, such as the calcium in bones, and aid metabolic functions, such as glucose metabolism.

Vitamins are carbon-containing compounds that enable many chemical reactions to occur in the body, some of which unlock the energy-yielding potential of carbohydrates, fats, proteins, and alcohol. Vitamins themselves provide no energy for the body.

A kcalorie is the amount of heat it takes to raise the temperature of 1 liter of water 1° C.

Organic compounds contain carbon atoms bonded to hydrogen atoms. Inorganic compounds lack carbon atoms bonded to hydrogen atoms. These terms have no relation to organic gardening.

Nutritional status is a measure of the extent to which a person is meeting his or her body's nutrient needs.

Dietary fiber consists of plant substances that are not digested by human enzymes in the intestinal tract. They then contribute to the bulk of the stool.

Based on nutrition surveys, name three nutrients that may be low in our diets.

Name four important factors that influence our food habits.

What is the approximate percent kcalorie breakdown of the U.S. diet in terms of carbohydrate, fat, and protein?

List the ABCD of nutrition assessment.

Define the word percent.

Represent the prefixes micro, milli, centi, and kilo by numbers.

Illustrate the conversion of a kilogram to pounds, an ounce to grams, a meter to inches, and an inch to centimeters.

A basic plan for health promotion and disease prevention includes which six parts?

Choose any four of: taste, habit, early experiences, routine, one's personal notion of good health, advertising, social factors, and economics.

Choose any of: iron, calcium, vitamin A, vitamin B-6, vitamin C, magnesium, and zinc. Dietary fiber is not a nutrient, but it is often poorly consumed as well.

<u>a</u>nthropometric

<u>b</u>iochemical

<u>c</u>linical

<u>d</u>ietary

14% to 16% of kcalories as protein,

44% to 47% of kcalories as carbohydrates,

35% to 38% of kcalories as fat.

micro = 1/1,000,000

milli = 1/1,000

centi = 1/100

kilo = 1,000

The term percent refers to a part of the total when the total represents 100 parts.

- Eat a healthful diet
- Exercise
- Don't smoke
- Limit alcohol intake
- Limit stress
- Consult health care professionals when necessary

1 kilogram = 2.2 pounds
1 ounce = 28 grams
1 meter = 39.4 inches
1 inch = 2.54 centimeters

CHAPTER 2

Define the term RDA.

What do these represent?

Define ESADDI.

Contrast biochemical versus clinical lesion.

If your dietary intake of vitamin C does not meet your RDA, does that mean you necessarily have a poor diet? Why?

Name the six exchange system groups.

What is an "exchange"?

Contrast malnutrition with overnutrition.

In what way is a food with a Standard of Identity excluded from current food labelling regulations?

ESADDI stands for the Estimated Safe and Adequate Daily Dietary Intake, set for several nutrients that have no true RDA. This includes copper, biotin, and chromium.

RDA stands for Recommended Dietary Allowance(s). These are set by the Food and Nutrition Board of the National Academy of Sciences and suggest the amount of a nutrient that should meet the needs of practically all healthy people.

The RDA reflects group -- not individual -- needs. You may need less than the RDA to maintain health. However, the further you stray from the RDA, the greater your risk for a nutritional deficiency.

A biochemical lesion is seen through an examination of blood or urine products, whereas a clinical lesion is seen on visual inspection of the body.

An "exchange" refers to a proper serving size for a food within an exchange group. For instance, one slice of bread is one starch/bread exchange, as is half a bagel.

Milk group
Fruit group
Vegetables group
Starch/bread group
Meat group
Fat group

They are foods that currently are excused from listing ingredients because they have followed a certain recipe that essentially remains the same from brand to brand.

Malnutrition simply represents poor nutrition. This could be due to an inadequate or excess nutrient intake. Overnutrition specifically refers to an excess of nutrient intake, such as when an excess kcalorie intake leads to obesity.

What is meant when a food is said to be nutrient dense?

Contrast the terms:

- positive balance

- negative balance

- equilibrium

Describe how the recommendations for energy and sodium intake differ from those for many vitamins.

What is the U.S. RDA?

How is it used?

How does it relate to the term Daily Values (DVs)?

Define the term essential nutrient.

Name four diseases the Dietary Guidelines are designed to help prevent.

Describe the current Food Guide Pyramid. What is its purpose?

What are three suggestions that can improve food choices made from the Food Guide Pyramid?

Positive balance refers to a greater consumption of a nutrient than is excreted, while negative balance is the opposite. In equilibrium consumption equals excretion.

Nutrient density reflects the nutrient content of food in relation to its kcalorie content. Nutrient-dense foods are rich in nutrients compared to kcalorie content.

The U.S. RDA exists in four versions. The adult version generally reflects the highest RDA value for persons in any age or gender category over age four years. The U.S. RDA is used on traditional nutrition labels. The new food labels will use another standard (Daily Values or DVs). The nutrients in a food are compared to this set standard.

The RDA for energy is based on average needs. The Food and Nutrition Board warns that the energy RDA is only a rough estimate, and intake should depend on activity. No RDA exists for sodium, only an estimate of a minimum requirement for health.

The Dietary Guidelines are designed to reduce the risk for chronic diseases, such as heart disease, hypertension, cancer, and cirrhosis of the liver.

An essential nutrient is a nutrient that cannot be manufactured by the body fast enough and therefore must be supplied in the diet.

1) Servings from the milk, yogurt, and cheese group should be low-fat or nonfat.
2) Some servings from beans, nuts, and seeds should be included.
3) Citrus fruits and dark green vegetables should be used.
4) Emphasis should be placed on whole-grain breads and cereals.

The Food Guide Pyramid has six groups: -milk, yogurt, and cheese; -meat, poultry, fish, dry beans, eggs, and nuts; -fruits, -vegetables; -breads, cereals, rice, and pasta; -fats, oils, and sweets. Consuming the recommended servings from each of these groups should supply nutrient needs.

What is the purpose of the Exchange System?

List the seven Dietary Guidelines.

Describe two major changes in the nutrient standards to be used on the new food labels.

List the adult servings from the Food Guide Pyramid.

Name two important nutrients found in each food group in the Food Guide Pyramid.

What is a risk associated with the use of health claims on labels?

What does the term "empty calorie" mean?

Explain the main difference between the U.S. RDAs and the new RDIs.

The Guidelines suggest one should eat a variety of foods; maintain healthy body weight; choose foods low in fat, saturated fat, and cholesterol; eat plenty of fruits, vegetables, and grains; choose foods low in salt and sugar; and use alcohol only in moderation, if at all.

The Exchange System arranges foods into six different categories that are designed so that, after noting the proper serving size, each food within a category provides about the same amount of carbohydrate, protein, fat, and kcalories.

2:	milk/yogurt/cheese
2 to 3:	meat/poultry/fish/beans/ eggs/nuts
2 to 3:	fruits
3 to 5:	vegetables
6 to 11:	breads/cereals/rice/ pasta
moderation:	fats/oils/sweets

On the new food labels, RDIs will replace the U.S. RDAs, and DRVs will be included for nutrients that do not have an RDA. Both will be combined into Daily Values expressed as a percentage of daily needs based on a 2,000 or 2,500 kcalorie diet.

The whole story may not be told. For example, the benefits from fiber in the food may not be balanced by the problems possible with high doses.

milk/yogurt/cheese: calcium, riboflavin
meat/poultry/fish/beans: protein, iron
fruits and vegetable groups: vitamins A
                                    and C
breads/cereals: thiamin, iron
fats/oils/sweets: essential fats,
                          vitamin E

The U.S. RDAs are based on the 1968 RDA and reflect percentages of the highest determined values. The name RDIs will soon replace the term U.S. RDAs.

A food that supplies kcalories, but offers little nutrient value is often referred to as an "empty calorie" food.

CHAPTER 3

Define the term quack.

Describe the term organically grown.

Name five beneficial qualities of a food additive.

Why is the term health food essentially misleading?

Are natural vitamins always superior to synthetic?

Are megadoses of vitamins generally healthful or harmful?

Define herbal therapy.

Define the term epidemiology.

Why is it used by some people?

Organic growers usually reject pesticides and use natural soil improvers, such as compost instead of chemical fertilizers. Also, crop rotation is used to further enrich soil and biological intervention is used to control pests.

A quack is a pretender of medical skills. He or she talks pretentiously without sound knowledge of the subject discussed.

Health food stores often suggest that some foods are "super nutrition foods." However, this is misleading because all foods eaten in moderation are healthy in the context of a balanced diet. As well, any food eaten in excess can be unhealthy.

Food additives often retard growth of microorganisms, prevent development of off-flavors, keep mixtures from separating, retain food crispiness, and may even raise the nutritional value.

A megadose of a vitamin is defined as an intake of quantities greater than 10 times the RDA. Though bodily chemical imbalances contribute to many diseases, meganutrient therapies have not been accepted as a remedy. Instead, these often cause harmful side effects.

No, the slightly different structure of a few synthetic vitamins does not decrease their value inside the body. Your body usually cannot tell a natural vitamin from a synthetic one. The main difference is the price: "natural" costs more.

Epidemiology is the study of disease patterns in specific populations. For instance, since the classical deficiency symptoms of pellagra appeared in only certain areas of the U.S., this suggested that a specific dietary factor in the diets of those individuals caused the disease.

Herbal therapy uses certain roots, plants, bark, and seeds as medical treatment. Scientific evidence shows that most herbal remedies lack effectiveness and in some cases are dangerous.

Name five ways to spot a quack.

Name two government agencies involved in prosecuting quackery.

Name two sources of reliable nutrition information.

Contrast hypothesis and theory.

How can freedom of speech and freedom of the press harm the consumer and protect the phony food promoter?

How do quacks find their victims?

Name four common sources of nutrition quackery.

Describe a double-blind experimental approach.

The Federal Trade Commission is one group which protects persons against false claims. Also, the Postal Service can act against persons making false claims for products sold through the mail.

Beware when promoters profess that: 1) particular foods can cure specific diseases; 2) only "natural" food should be eaten; 3) modern processing methods strip the nutrition value from foods; 4) sugar is a deadly poison; 5) stress greatly increases your need for nutrients.

A hypothesis is a possible explanation of an event from which to base an experiment. A theory is an idea that is supported by multiple lines of research, or in other words, many hypotheses that have proven true.

Physicians and Registered Dietitians are reliable sources of nutrition information.

The important aspect of their success is marketing "tender loving care". Clients often praise the people at the health food store because they take time to share "interesting" discoveries in the health field.

Though it would be illegal to label a vitamin as a cure for cancer, if one falsely promotes a product but is not the actual vendor, one cannot be charged. Retailers often rely on talk shows or magazine articles to provide the misinformation they need to sell their products.

A double-blind experiment tests a hypothesis in a way that neither the subjects nor the researchers know which subjects are receiving the experimental treatment (such as supplemental vitamins) and which subjects are receiving the placebo-- "fake" medicine. The code is broken only after the experiment is over.

1)   radio
2)   television
3)   newspapers
4)   books and magazines

CHAPTER 4

Define the term active absorption.

What is required for it?

What is the life span of a typical absorptive cell?

What does a life span of that magnitude represent in terms of nutrient needs?

Define the term ulcer.

What are two good preventive measures for limiting the risk of developing an ulcer?

What is the key factor that aids absorption of nutrients in the small intestine?

Define the term transit time.

What is a typical transit time?

If a person has heartburn, what is a likely cause?

How is the lymphatic system important to nutrition?

Name one or more enzymes that act on the following substances:

proteins
triglycerides
sucrose
lactose
amylose

The life span of an absorptive cell is about 2 to 5 days. Such a rapid cell turnover puts great demands on the body for nutrients, such as protein, vitamin A, vitamin C, folate, and zinc.

Active absorption represents absorbing a compound from a low concentration into a high concentration. It requires the expenditure of energy and a carrier molecule.

The key factor is the villi, finger-like projections that extend into the intestine and create a large surface area for absorption.

An ulcer is an erosion into the tissue of the stomach or small intestine. The best way to limit the risk for an ulcer is 1) don't smoke cigarettes, and 2) don't abuse aspirin, alcohol, or other factors that reduce the health of cells of the GI tract.

Overeating, especially lying down after a large meal, is a likely cause. A full stomach tends to force food up through the lower esophageal sphincter into the esophagus, where the acid chyme irritates the esophagus, causing heartburn.

Transit time refers to the period required for a meal to traverse the gastrointestinal tract. This normally takes 1 to three days. Faster rates are seen in people who consume adequate fiber.

proteins	-	pepsin, trypsin
triglycerides	-	lipase
sucrose	-	sucrase
lactose	-	lactase
amylose	-	amylase

The lymphatic vessels that serve the small intestine pick up the products of fat absorption and deliver them to the bloodstream. These substances are too large to enter the bloodstream directly.

Indicate the sites of enzyme production in the GI tract and its accessory organs.

List and give examples of the sequence from cells to organism as biological complexity increases in the body.

How efficient is digestion and absorption of food?

What are hemorrhoids and how do they occur?

Describe the role of saliva in digestion.

Describe the major role of the colon.

List the major substances absorbed in the stomach, small intestine, and large intestine (colon).

Name four hormones that influence nutrient use in the body and their main functions.

1.) cells -   basic unit of life.
2.) tissues - bone, cartilage, muscle, nerve.
3.) organs - skin, kidney, liver.
4.) organ system - digestive, respiratory system
5.) organism - human body

Enzymes are produced in the mouth, stomach, pancreas, and the wall of the small intestine.

Hemorrhoids are swollen veins of the rectum and anus caused by added stress from pregnancy, obesity, prolonged sitting, violent coughing or sneezing, or straining during elimination.

About 90% to 95% of all food substances are digested and absorbed. Little protein, carbohydrate, or fat is excreted in the feces.

The major role of the colon is to finish the absorption of water and minerals from the diet, and thus prepare the feces for elimination. Most water and minerals in the diet, however, are absorbed in the small intestine.

Saliva is secreted by glands in the mouth. It contains mucus that envelops and lubricates chewed foods, facilitating passage down the GI tract. Saliva also contains enzymes that break down carbohydrates into smaller units.

---

insulin -   regulates blood glucose and hunger.
thyroid hormones - regulate metabolic rate.
gastrin -   regulate stomach's digestive processes.
secretin -   acts on pancreas and gallbladder.

---

stomach -- some alcohol
small intestine -- peptides and amino acids; monosaccharides (single sugars); monoglycerides and free fatty acids; vitamins; minerals; and water
large intestine -- some minerals, water, and fiber by-products

Provide four suggestions for someone who commonly develops constipation.

Name the major parts of the GI tract and its related organs.

In what organ does most digestion and absorption occur?

Define the term enzyme and describe the role enzymes play in digestion.

Define the term passive absorption. What nutrient is absorbed this way?

In consecutive order, name the parts of the GI tract from mouth to anus.

List two ways in which a laxative works. Are they always safe to use?

Define the term villi and describe their function in the small intestine.

The GI tract includes the mouth, stomach, small intestine, large intestine, and anus. Entering into the small intestine are the pancreas and the liver (the latter via the gallbladder).

1) Increase intake of food fibers, such as bran fiber, which draw more water into the intestine, thus easing elimination of the stool.
2) Drink adequate water.
3) Eat dried fruits.
4) Perform regular exercise.

Enzymes speed reaction rates. In digestion, enzymes such as pepsin speed the breakdown of food products into the basic components that can be absorbed by the body.

Much digestion and absorption occur in the small intestine, specifically in the duodenum and upper half of the jejunum.

mouth

esophagus

stomach

small intestine

large intestine

rectum

anus

Passive absorption is that which requires permeability of the substance through the wall of the small intestine, as well as a higher concentration of the substance in the small intestine than in the absorptive cells.

Fats are absorbed this way.

Villi are finger-like protrusions in the small intestine. They participate in the digestion and absorption of foodstuffs, mostly by increasing the surface area of the intestinal tract.

Laxatives work by 1) irritating the intestinal nerve junctions or
2) drawing water into the intestine to enlarge the stool.

No, with regular use they can decrease muscle action in the large intestine, causing more constipation.

If a person experiences malabsorption of carbohydrate, how will he or she be affected?

Describe those consequences.

Relate sugar intake to dental caries.

Contrast hyperglycemia and hypoglycemia.

What are ketones, and how are they linked to a low-carbohydrate diet?

What is the main function for carbohydrate in the body, and for what two types of cells is this function most evident?

Describe why carbohydrates are "protein sparing."

What is phenylketonuria?

Link it to aspartame (NutraSweet).

Define the term disaccharide and give two examples.

Bacteria on the teeth metabolize sugars into acids that can dissolve the tooth enamel, thus leading to dental caries.

Unabsorbed nutrients that make their way into the large intestine stimulate bacterial growth there. This results in the production of acids and gasses, which cause abdominal bloating and discomfort.

Ketones are produced from breakdown products of fatty acids. When insufficient carbohydrate is consumed, fat metabolism is inhibited. The byproducts of fat metabolism build up in the liver, which converts these into ketones.

Hyperglycemia means high glucose levels in the bloodstream.

Hypoglycemia means low glucose in the bloodstream.

Cells need glucose for energy production. If you do not eat glucose, the body is forced to synthesize glucose from other nutrients, mainly the amino acids that make up proteins. Carbohydrates in the diet "spare" protein from this use.

Carbohydrate is mainly used for energy production in cells, especially in <u>brain cells</u> and <u>red blood cells</u>. These cells have a poor ability to metabolize other energy-yielding substances.

Disaccharide means double sugar (di- means two). Examples are sucrose -- formed from glucose plus fructose; lactose -- formed from glucose plus galactose; maltose -- formed from two glucose molecules bonded together.

In phenylketonuria (PKU) a person's liver has a reduced ability to metabolize the amino acid phenylalanine. Since aspartame contains phenylalanine, people with PKU should not use products containing aspartame.

What is the structure of aspartame, and what are two of its characteristics?

Define the term monosaccharide and provide two examples.

Define the term polysaccharide and provide two examples.

Define the term dietary fiber and provide three examples.

Relate the terms fiber and diverticula.

Name the two types of diabetes and their typical causes.

Compare the benefits of soluble and insoluble dietary fibers on the body.

Name two food sources of each.

How much carbohydrate must one eat each day to avoid ketosis?

Monosaccharide means single sugar (mono- stands for one). Examples are glucose, fructose, and galactose.

Aspartame is made of two amino acids and a methanol molecule; therefore, it is not a carbohydrate, but a protein. It is about 200 times sweeter than sucrose. Aspartame still provides kcalories (4 kcalories per gram), but is so sweet that little is needed.

Dietary fiber refers to foodstuffs that are not digested by human enzymes in the intestinal tract. These include cellulose, hemicellulose, pectins, gums, and mucilages.

Poly means many, so polysaccharides have many sugar units. Amylose is a straight-chain polysaccharide, also called starch.

Glycogen is animal starch and is highly branched.

Insulin-dependent diabetes usually develops in childhood and results from immune system destruction of the insulin-producing cells in the pancreas. Noninsulin-dependent diabetes usually develops in adulthood and is often caused by obesity. Large fat cells are not very sensitive to insulin.

Fiber makes a softer and larger stool which then decreases pressures inside the large intestine during defecation. If a low-fiber diet is consumed, the pressures may be high, causing small pouches called diverticula to pop out in the large intestine wall.

Consuming 50 to 100 grams of carbohydrate a day should prevent ketosis. This amount of carbohydrate should allow for complete fat metabolism.

Soluble dietary fibers found in oats and beans are associated with the lowering of blood glucose and blood cholesterol levels. Insoluble fibers, found in wheat bran and popcorn, are primarily associated with increased fecal bulk and, in turn, less constipation.

What are three dietary recommendations for a person who has hypoglycemia?

What are two possible problems resulting from consuming a diet too high in dietary fiber?

Provide some suggestions for a person with lactose intolerance.

Besides reducing diverticulosis, can dietary fiber prevent any other diseases?

What do the Dietary Guidelines suggest as food choices to encourage an ample carbohydrate intake?

How much fiber should one eat?

Compare the terms soluble and insoluble fiber, especially in terms of their digestibility.

Name three hormones that help regulate blood glucose levels. Indicate the effect of each.

Very high dietary fiber intakes, such as 60 grams per day, may cause a very large stool that is hard to eliminate and may bind up important minerals, such as calcium, zinc, and iron. In a child's diet the bulkiness of fiber foods may make it difficult to consume enough kcalories.

A person with hypoglycemia should:

1) consume meals on a regular basis

2) have some protein in each meal

3) have a moderate simple sugar intake

Dietary fiber intake can be used to control blood glucose and cholesterol levels and possibly reduce the risk of colon cancer.

If the person still wants to consume milk products he can eat smaller portions, yogurt (which supplies its own lactase), cheese (which is naturally low in lactose), and drink milk in which the lactose has already been converted into glucose and galactose.

A reasonable goal is 10 to 13 grams per 1,000 kcalories, or up to 35 grams of fiber per day.

The Dietary Guidelines suggest increasing the intake of carbohydrates in the forms of fruits, vegetables, and grains.

When hyperglycemia develops, insulin attempts to lower blood glucose levels. When hypoglycemia develops, glucagon, epinephrine, and other hormones break down glycogen in the liver to raise blood glucose levels.

Insoluble fibers neither dissolve in water, nor are metabolized by intestinal bacteria. They include cellulose, hemicellulose, and lignins. Soluble fibers either dissolve in water or swell when put into water. They include pectins, gums, and mucilages.

CHAPTER 6

Name the two essential fatty acids.

What are their structures?

Contrast the term lipids with the term fats and oils.

What functions do eicosanoids perform?

What is the current American Heart Association (AHA) recommendation for fat intake?

Contrast omega-3 and omega-6 fatty acids based on their effects on blood clotting.

Name the site where essentially all digestion and absorption of lipids takes place.

What are the five most important risk factors for heart disease?

List three changes a person can make to lower a high serum cholesterol level.

Which is the most important change to make?

Lipids include all compounds that dissolve in ether, and chloroform. Fats are lipids that are solid at room temperature, and oils are lipids that are liquid at room temperature.

| Linoleic acid - | 18 carbon atoms, 2 double bonds, omega-6. |
| Linolenic acid - | 18 carbon atoms, 3 double bonds, omega-3. The alpha form is the most important. |

The AHA recommends that a diet contain no more than 30% of total kcalories as fat, with a ratio of 1:1:1 (10% of kcalories each) each of saturated fat, monounsaturated fat, and polyunsaturated fat.

Eicosanoids help control blood clotting, and inflammatory responses in the body.

Small intestine.

When the body synthesizes eicosanoids from omega-3 fatty acids, these tend to decrease blood clotting and inflammatory processes; eicosanoids from the omega-6 fatty acids generally increase these processes.

1) Reduce saturated fat intake. This is the most important change to make.

2) Reduce cholesterol intake

3) Increase intake of soluble fiber

1) Smoking
2) Hypertension (high blood pressure)
3) High serum LDL-cholesterol levels
4) Diabetes
5) Advancing age

Describe the route that most dietary fats take through the body to arrive at an adipose cell.

What is a phospholipid?

Give an example.

What is the current serum cholesterol cut-off level for institution of diet therapy?

Name four functions of fat.

Advertisers tout certain brands of peanut butter as having no cholesterol. Is there something unique about these brands of peanut butter?

Differentiate between the absorption paths followed by long-chain fatty acids versus those taken by short- and medium-chain fatty acids.

What is cholesterol?

How do we obtain cholesterol?

What are two things it does?

Define the term triglyceride.

Where are these found?

A phospholipid is a compound with a triglyceride-like structure, but which has only one or two fatty acids. The other sites on the glycerol are bonded to something other than fatty acids; a phosphate group can be part of the additional structure. A common example is lecithin.

Most dietary fats, being long-chained, are absorbed into the intestinal cells and formed into chylomicrons. These travel through the lymphatic system into the bloodstream. The fat is then extracted using the enzyme lipoprotein lipase from the chylomicron and is absorbed into cells.

Fat is used for:

1) energy storage,
2) providing energy to the body,
3) providing satiety,
4) insulating and protecting the body,
5) transporting fat-soluble vitamins
    during absorption from the intestine,
6) providing flavor and texture to food,
7) forming eicosanoids.

200 milligrams of cholesterol per 100 milliliters (dl) of serum.

Note: dl = deciliter
       deci = 1/10 or 10^{-1}

Long-chain fatty acids travel from the small intestine into the lymphatic system, from there they enter the bloodstream.

Short- and medium-chain fatty acids enter directly from the small intestine into the portal vein, from there they travel to the liver.

No, since no plant food has cholesterol. No peanut butter would contain cholesterol if it were made free of animal products.

Triglyceride refers to a structure with a three carbon glycerol backbone and three fatty acids attached to the glycerol. Triglycerides are the major form of fat in food and in the body.

Cholesterol is a multi-ringed, waxy substance. Our cells make cholesterol, and we consume it in foods. It is formed into parts of 1) cell membranes, and 2) various hormones and other body structures.

Define the term rancid.

What is nature's natural protection against rancidity?

What is so special about fish oils?

Define the term hydrogenation, and explain why this process is used in foods.

How much fat does one need to consume? Why?

Define the term bile and its role in digestion and absorption.

What are two symptoms of an essential fatty acid deficiency?

Contrast the receptor pathway versus the scavenger pathway for LDL uptake.

Define the term emulsifier.

What do these do?

Fish oils contain a high percentage of omega-3 fatty acids, especially EPA and DHA. These compounds at low doses tend to reduce blood clotting, and at high doses can reduce levels of triglycerides and cholesterol in the bloodstream (but especially triglycerides).

Rancidity reflects the breakdown of polyunsaturated fats at the double bonds. Nature provides vitamin E to protect against the breakdown of the double bonds in a fatty acid, and therefore reduce rancidity. In this case vitamin E acts as an antioxidant.

One needs to consume approximately 1 tablespoon of vegetable oils per day to obtain the essential fatty acids. These essential fatty acids are necessary for synthesizing eicosanoids.

Hydrogenation refers to the adding of hydrogen atoms to the carbon-carbon double bonds of fatty acids. This turns liquid oils into solid fats and therefore creates margarines and shortenings that are ideal for making some foods, such as pastries and frostings.

Flaky skin and diarrhea often develop during essential fatty acid deficiency.

Bile, made by the liver and secreted by the gallbladder, breaks large fat globules into tiny droplets. This increases the surface area for enzyme action and ends up speeding fat digestion by lipase enzymes.

An emulsifier, such as bile or lecithin, suspends fat in water, as when lecithin suspends fat in the watery chyme during digestion. In essence, droplets of fat become surrounded by shells of water.

In the receptor pathway, _body cells_ recognize LDL in the bloodstream, take it up, digest it, and use its parts. In the scavenger pathway, _white blood cells_ buried in blood vessels pick up LDL particles and take these up, in turn allowing cholesterol and other fats to invade the blood vessel wall.

Contrast omega-3 with omega-6 fatty acids with regards to structure.

What is the "good" cholesterol and the "bad" cholesterol?

Is "bad" cholesterol all bad?

Contrast saturated, monounsaturated, and polyunsaturated fatty acids.

Describe the route of cholesterol synthesized by the liver as it travels from there to cells in the body.

What is an antioxidant?

How does one work?

How does chain length and degree of saturation of fatty acids affect the solid or liquid nature of lipids?

What is a chylomicron?

Define its role in the body.

What is the current recommendation for fish and fish oil intake?

HDL is the "good" cholesterol as it encourages cholesterol loss from cells. LDL cholesterol is the "bad" version since it takes cholesterol to cells. However, LDL is only "bad" when it is at high levels since it also serves a vital role in the body. Cells need some cholesterol to function.

Omega-3 fatty acids have the first double bond after the third carbon from the methyl (CH_3) end, whereas omega-6 fatty acids have the first double bond after the sixth carbon from the methyl end.

Cholesterol synthesized by the liver is incorporated into a very low density lipoprotein (VLDL). This turns into a low density lipoprotein (LDL) in the bloodstream. Then cells take up the LDLs, and by doing that the cholesterol in the LDLs.

<u>Saturated</u> fatty acids contain <u>no</u> C=C double bonds in their structure.

<u>Monounsaturated</u> fatty acids contain <u>one</u> C=C double bond.

<u>Polyunsaturated</u> fatty acids contain <u>two or more</u> C=C double bonds.

Long chain length and saturated fatty acids produce solid fats, whereas polyunsaturated fatty acids always produce liquid oils. Note that a short chain length overrides the effects of saturation and produces a liquid oil, even if the fatty acids are saturated, as in coconut oil.

An antioxidant is a compound that stops oxidizing agents from taking electrons from compounds. For lipids, antioxidants protect the double bonds present by donating electrons to electron-seeking compounds. Vitamin E is a natural antioxidant.

Eating fish once or twice a week is a good dietary practice to obtain omega-3 fatty acids. Fish oil capsules are not recommended, unless under a physician's guidance.

A chylomicron is a droplet of fat surrounded by a shell of protein and various specialized fats. The chylomicron structure allows fat to travel in the water base of the bloodstream; therefore, cells that need the fat have access to it via the bloodstream.

CHAPTER 7

How do proteins specifically contribute to maintaining fluid balance?

How is this linked to edema?

To what does the term complementary proteins refer?

Name four functions of protein in the body.

Describe the "all-or-none" law with regard to amino acid metabolism.

What is the relationship between nitrogen and protein?

Contrast high quality (complete) and low quality (incomplete) proteins.

Name two food sources for each type.

What characteristic does the order of the amino acids give to a protein?

What is the Recommended Dietary Allowance (RDA) for protein for a 154-pound (70-kilogram) man?

When one food protein makes up for the lack of an amino acid in another food protein, the two proteins are said to complement each other; one protein complements the weakness in the other.

Blood proteins counteract the force of blood pressure. As blood pressure tries to force fluid out of the bloodstream, proteins act to attract the fluid back. If insufficient protein is in the bloodstream, excessive fluid leaks out into the tissue spaces; this can lead to edema.

The "all-or-none" law states that if all essential amino acids are not available for synthesizing needed proteins, the amino acids present cannot be used at that time. Thus protein synthesis will not occur.

Proteins 1) produce vital body constituents, such as muscles and blood clotting factors. Proteins also help 2) maintain fluid balance, 3) maintain acid base balance, form hormones and enzymes, contribute to immune function, 4) form glucose when needed, and 5) provide energy for the body.

High quality (complete) proteins contain all nine essential amino acids, whereas low quality (incomplete) proteins lack sufficient amounts of all essential amino acids.

All proteins contain nitrogen, on average 16% nitrogen. Therefore, nitrogen (in grams) times 6.25 = protein (in grams). The same holds if nitrogen is divided by 0.16.

In the United States the RDA for protein is 0.8 grams per kilogram of body weight. So 70 x 0.8 = 56 grams of protein.

The order of the amino acids in a protein determines the function of the protein, since it dictates its three-dimensional shape.

What does denature represent in terms of a protein?

Define the term amino acid, and contrast essential amino acid with nonessential amino acid.

Describe three types of vegetarianism.

Relate the terms <u>positive</u>, <u>negative</u>, and <u>equilibrium</u> to protein balance.

Contrast kwashiorkor and marasmus.

List the major sites of protein digestion and absorption in the body.

Describe the danger associated with amino acid supplementation.

What is meant by the term limiting amino acid.

An amino acid is a compound with a central carbon atom. Linked to it is an acid group, a hydrogen atom, an amine-group, and another chemical group that gives the amino acid its identity. Essential amino acids must be present in the diet. Nonessential amino acids can be made by the body.

If the three-dimensional structure of a protein is destroyed by acid or alkaline solutions, agitation, heat, or other processes, this is called denaturation of the protein.

In positive protein balance one would be gaining protein tissue, such as in growth or during pregnancy. Negative protein balance refers to a loss of protein tissue, such as seen in starvation or illness. Protein equilibrium refers to body maintenance, as in adulthood.

Vegans are total vegetarians and eat only plant foods. Fruitarians eat primarily fruits, nuts, honey, and vegetable oils. Both need to ensure some food they eat is fortified with vitamin B-12. Lactovegetarians add dairy products. Lacto-ovo-vegetarians add dairy products and eggs.

digestion: stomach
              small intestine

absorption: small intestine

Kwashiorkor is a disease that primarily effects young children who are already ill and follow a diet poor in kcalories, especially one poor in protein. The child develops edema but has fat stores.

Marasmus develops in infants from essentially a starvation diet, grossly inadequate in both proteins and kcalories. The infant does not show edema and has little or no fat stores.

The essential amino acid in shortest supply in a food or diet limits the amount of protein the body can synthesize.

Amino acid supplements may trigger imbalances in the body which occur because chemically similar amino acids compete for absorption into the blood. An excess of one can create high demand for a carrier and hamper the absorption of another amino acid.

What is the name for the niacin deficiency disease, and what are two of its symptoms?

List two functions of vitamin D.

What is a vitamin?

Can high intakes of water-soluble vitamins be harmful?

If so, which two vitamins are examples?

Provide one example of how vitamins A, D, E, and K are different from the other vitamins?

List two ways water-soluble vitamins are lost in cooking.

Define the term coenzyme.

Name two of the best food sources of riboflavin.

What is our main food source?

Vitamin D helps regulate absorption of calcium and phosphorus and the deposition of calcium in bones.

Pellagra is caused by a prolonged niacin deficiency. Symptoms include the four "D"s -- diarrhea, dermatitis, dementia, and death.

When taken in large doses (more than 100 times the RDA) water-soluble vitamins can be toxic, especially vitamin B-6 and niacin.

Vitamins are carbon-containing (organic) compounds needed by the body via diet in small amounts for important metabolic reactions.

Water-soluble vitamins are easily lost in cooking because of heat, alkalinity, and leaching into the cooking water.

Vitamins A, D, E, and K are fat-soluble, whereas the B vitamins and vitamin C dissolve in water.

Liver, mushrooms, spinach, and milk are the most nutrient-dense sources of riboflavin. Milk products are our major food contributors.

Coenzymes are structures that directly help enzymes function.

Name two nutrient-dense sources of niacin and a component in food that can form niacin.

Do nutrition experts recommend general use of a vitamin and mineral supplement?

What is one function of pantothenic acid?

List two good food sources of thiamin.

What is the main function of biotin? Name two sources.

What is a key guideline to use when choosing a vitamin supplement?

What is the most important function of vitamin B-6?

What is the term for a thiamin deficiency?

What body functions quickly show signs of it?

No, nutrition experts believe that a diet following the Food Guide Pyramid provides a diet sufficient in vitamins and minerals for most healthy persons.

Mushrooms, wheat bran, tuna and other fish, chicken, asparagus, and peanuts are good sources. Each 60 milligrams of dietary tryptophan remaining after protein synthesis forms 1 milligram of niacin.

Foods containing a very high nutrient density of thiamin are pork products and sunflower seeds. Other good sources include whole grains, green beans, and organ meats.

Pantothenic acid allows many important energy-yielding reactions to take place, such as in glucose and fat metabolism.

A supplement should contain no more than 50% to 150% of the adult RDA for vitamins.

Biotin acts as a coenzyme in fat and carbohydrate by adding carbon dioxide to other compounds. Sources include cauliflower, egg yolk, cheese, liver, and intestinal synthesis by bacteria.

Beriberi is the name of the thiamin deficiency disease. Brain and nerve action suffer in a thiamin deficiency.

Protein metabolism is the most important function of vitamin B-6.

Is it necessary to obtain all vitamins daily?

List two functions of vitamin A.

Why are fat-soluble vitamins potentially harmful, and which are especially toxic?

Besides preformed vitamin A, in what other form does vitamin A activity exist in the diet?

Give three examples of people who may need to use vitamin and mineral supplements.

Relate a deficiency of vitamin E to a typical result, the breakdown of red blood cells.

List two good food sources of vitamin D.

Explain the role of the intrinsic factor in vitamin B-12 absorption.

Vitamin A functions to:
1) maintain vision.

2) ensure the health of the immune system.

3) direct aspects of growth and development.

Ideally, vitamins in food should be consumed daily, but an occasional lapse of intake for even the water-soluble vitamins is not harmful.

Potential vitamin A is present as the common plant pigments called carotenes or carotenoids.

The fat-soluble vitamins are poorly excreted and thus can reach toxic levels in the body, especially vitamins A and D.

A deficiency of vitamin E causes the breakdown (hemolysis) of red blood cells, especially in infancy. Vitamin E protects the polyunsaturated fatty acids and vitamin A in the cell membrane from destruction.

Vitamin and mineral supplementation should be considered for:
1) women with excessive during menses (iron), 2) pregnant and breast-feeding women (iron, folate), 3) total vegetarians (vitamin B-12, iron, calcium, zinc, others), 4) breast-fed infants (iron, vitamin D, and possibly fluoride).

The intrinsic factor (IF), a protein produced in the stomach, binds to vitamin B-12 in the small intestine. IF is necessary for the adequate absorption of vitamin B-12 in the ileum.

Good food sources of vitamin D include: fish oils, fatty fish, and fortified milk.

Name two good food sources of
vitamin B-6.

What are three main functions of
vitamin C?

What is the main danger of vitamin B-6
toxicity?

Name three nutrients linked to a
reduction in cancer?

How do they act?

What is the most important function of
folate?

What are two nutrient-dense sources of
folate?

Why does a folate deficiency lead to
anemia?

Why does FDA limit the amount of
folate allowed in a vitamin supplement?

Vitamin C is important for wound healing, enhancing iron absorption, and acting as an antioxidant.

Meats, fish, and poultry are the best sources, since the vitamin B-6 present in animal foods is better absorbed than that in plant foods.

Nutrients such as beta-carotene, vitamin E, vitamin C, and selenium have potential anticancer properties. They all act as part of antioxidant systems or are antioxidants themselves.

Irreversible nerve damage can result from intakes of 2 to 6 grams of vitamin B-6 per day for 2 to 40 months.

Green leafy vegetables, organ meats, sprouts, and orange juice are the best folate sources.

Folate is necessary for cell division because it contributes to the formation of DNA and RNA.

Excess folate intake can mask the early warning signs of a B-12 deficiency, a potentially dangerous condition necessitating early treatment.

In a folate deficiency, red blood cells can continue to produce enough protein to grow, but they cannot synthesize enough DNA to divide. The resulting large immature cells lead to a reduction in oxygen-carrying capacity of the blood, in part caused by a reduced life span of the cells. Thus, anemia results.

What is the main function of vitamin K?

Describe how an antioxidant functions.

List three good food sources of vitamin A.

Define xerophthalmia.

At what level of intake is vitamin A considered potentially toxic?

Name two nutrient-dense food sources of vitamin E.

Briefly describe the three stages of the cancer process.

What are three dietary recommendations to reduce the risk of cancer?

An antioxidant, such as vitamin E, donates electrons to an electron-seeking compound, in turn neutralizing it. This then protects other molecules from attack by the electron-seeking compounds.

Vitamin K is essential for blood clotting because it helps impart a calcium-binding ability to certain blood proteins.

Xerophthalmia, literally "dry eye," is a disease process initiated by a prolonged vitamin A deficiency in which the mucus-forming cells in the eye no longer function properly. Blindness eventually can result.

Foods with the highest nutrient density for vitamin A are carrots, liver, spinach and other greens, sweet potatoes, and yellow squash.

The best sources of vitamin E are plant oils, margarine, and asparagus.

Toxicity symptoms from excessive vitamin A intake are apparent with long-term supplement use at only five to ten times the RDA, especially during pregnancy.

Avoid obesity, reduce fat intake to less than 30% of total kcalories, eat more high fiber foods, eat foods rich in vitamins A and C, avoid excessive amounts of alcohol and use moderation when consuming cured foods.

initiation - chemicals, radiation, or viruses alter DNA.
promotion - alcohol, estrogen, dietary fat encourage division of altered cells.
progression - the ball of cells, or the developing cancerous tumor grows and invades surrounding tissues, eventually reaching lymph and blood vessels.

CHAPTER 9

Define the term bioavailability.

What is a potential danger from taking mineral supplements?

What two nonmineral substances can affect the bioavailability of minerals?

Name three excellent sources of iron.

What major role does water play in chemical reactions?

Contrast major and trace minerals.

Contrast the absorption rates for heme and nonheme iron.

Contrast the occurrence of iron deficiency and iron-deficiency anemia.

An excess intake of one mineral can influence the absorption and metabolism of other minerals; for example, a high zinc intake reduces copper absorption.

Bioavailability refers to the body's ability to absorb a nutrient from the diet.

Spinach, oysters, liver, clams, peas, and legumes are the most nutrient-dense sources of iron. Beef is also a good source.

Phytic acid in grain fibers and oxalic acid in leafy vegetables can both bind minerals and greatly decrease their absorption.

Major mineral needs are $\geq$ 100 milligrams per day; trace mineral needs are < 100 milligrams per day.

Water serves as a medium for chemical reactions. It also actively participates in some chemical reactions.

More people have low iron stores (about 30% of American women), than have overt iron-deficiency anemia.

Heme iron is absorbed more than twice as efficiently as nonheme iron, about 20% versus 2% to 10%.

Name two groups that are at risk for iron deficiency?   Why?

Name two food sources of copper.

What is a function of manganese in the body?

What is the effect on copper status of excessive use of zinc supplements?

What are two food sources of fluoride?

Name and describe a condition that results from prolonged iodide deficiency.

What is the most important function of chromium?

Name two sources of selenium for a diet.

Copper is primarily found in liver, cocoa, legumes, and whole grains.

Infants, preschoolers, adolescents, menstruating women, and pregnant women are at risk for iron deficiency, since their iron needs often exceed their usual iron intake.

Since copper and zinc compete with one another for absorption, overzealous supplementation of zinc can result in a copper deficiency.

Manganese is a component of many different enzymes, such as those used in carbohydrate metabolism, and is important in bone formation.

A goiter develops in an iodide deficiency as the thyroid gland enlarges, attempting to take up more iodide from the bloodstream. The growth failure and mental retardation associated with cretinism occurs in infants whose mothers had iodide-deficient diets during pregnancy.

Tea, seafood, and seaweed are the only good food sources of fluoride.

Fish, meats, organ meats, eggs, shellfish, and grains grown in selenium-rich soil are good food sources.

Chromium aids glucose uptake by the cells.

Estimate the fluid needs of an adult.

Name a function of fluoride in the body.

Compare the calcium intake of women over age 25 to their RDA for calcium.

Why is sodium's presence in the diet not a problem for everyone?

Describe the mechanism that limits iron absorption when iron stores are adequate.

What piece of advice should be given to the general public concerning prevention of hypertension?

Name three food sources of phosphorus in the diet.

Name the two good sources of iodide.

During teeth and bone development, fluoride allows for the production of tougher tooth crystals, which are more resistant to acid erosion.

Water needs for an adult can be roughly estimated as 1 milliliter per kcalorie of energy expended.

Only some persons are susceptible to sodium-linked hypertension. Even among people with hypertension, only part of this is caused by an excessive sodium intake.

The RDA for calcium is 800 milligrams, whereas the average calcium intake of women ranges from 500 to 650 milligrams. About 25% of women consume less than 300 milligrams daily.

To limit the risk of hypertension, consume a diet based on the Food Guide Pyramid, whole grains, fruits, and vegetables. This provides ample potassium, calcium, and magnesium, and a moderate amount of sodium. In addition, do not become obese.

The serum protein that carries iron is full when iron stores are adequate. This limits transfer of iron absorbed into intestinal cells to the bloodstream. This iron is then likely to be sloughed off with the intestinal cells and excreted.

Saltwater fish, seafood, plants grown near the sea, and iodized salt are the best sources of iodide.

Milk, cheese, bakery products, and meat provide most of the phosphorus in the diet.

Name three functions of magnesium.

How can young women attempt to limit their future risk for osteoporosis?

Name three food sources of magnesium in the diet.

Name two functions of phosphorus.

What are the two major functions of sodium?

Name two major functions of chloride.

Compare the amount of sodium added in food processing to that added during cooking and at mealtimes.

How are copper metabolism and iron metabolism related?

Young women can limit their future risk for osteoporosis by:

1) consuming the RDA for calcium
2) performing regular exercise
3) maintaining regular menses
4) moderating tobacco and alcohol use, if applicable.

Magnesium is an important cofactor for more than 300 enzymes. Proper nerve and cardiac functions require magnesium.

Phosphorus is a component of enzymes, ATP, cell membranes, and the bone.

Whole grains, broccoli, squash, bran, nuts, and seeds are excellent magnesium sources. The best sources are plant products.

Chloride forms a negative ion that is an important part of extracellular fluid. These ions also are part of stomach acid and are used during immune responses.

Sodium is the major positive ion of extracellular fluid and is partly responsible for fluid balance in this and other compartments. Sodium is also important in nerve cell conduction.

A copper-containing protein aids in release of iron from storage. Copper deficiency can lead to an iron deficiency.

Approximately 1/3 to 1/2 of the sodium in the diet is added in cooking or at the table. One half is a result of manufacturing procedures. Very little occurs naturally in foods.

Name three major functions of zinc in the body.

Name three good food sources of zinc.

Compare the minimum requirement for sodium to our average daily intakes.

Name three major functions of calcium in the body.

Where is most of the potassium found in the body? Name two functions of this mineral.

Compare the composition of healthy bone versus bone in osteoporotic people.

Is this the same difference as seen between rickets and osteomalacia?

Name three good food sources of potassium.

Name three major contributors of calcium in the diet.

Oysters, shellfish, beef, and turkey are rich in zinc. Generally, protein-rich foods are good sources of zinc.

Major functions of zinc include DNA and protein metabolism, wound healing, growth, vitamin A mobilization, proper immune function, and proper development of sexual organs and bones.

Calcium is essential for bone health, blood clotting, muscle contraction, and nerve transmission.

The minimum requirement for sodium is 500 milligrams daily, whereas the average American intake is more than 6 times that, 3 to 7 grams daily. That is equivalent to 7.5 to 18 grams of salt daily.

The bone composition in osteoporosis is essentially the same as normal bone; however, less total bone exists throughout the body.

No, bone in rickets and osteomalacia has decreased calcium composition compared to normal bone.

Almost all the potassium in the body is in the intracellular fluid. Its functions are analogous to those of sodium, namely fluid balance and nerve transmission.

Dairy products such as milk and cheese provide most of the calcium in the diet. White bread and rolls also are contributors.

Fruits, vegetables, milk, whole grains, and meats are all good potassium sources.

CHAPTER 10

List three reasons why the body resists weight loss.

Is there any evidence to support the idea that eating meat and potatoes will stop the digestion of both foods, or that one should consume exclusively fresh fruits before noon, as some fad diet books suggest?

Why is weight loss generally so rapid in the first week of the diet?

Why should the prevention of obesity be emphasized?

Losing about 1 to 2 pounds of weight per week is typically a goal of sound weight loss plans.

Justify that recommendation for the rate of weight loss.

What is the three-pronged approach that a well-designed diet should take?

What are the best foods to consume when trying to lose weight?

What is the lowest kcalorie consumption per day that still allows for an adequate diet?

None that I can think of.

This is pure nonsense.

1)	Thyroid hormone levels, and so basal metabolism, drop.
2)	The fat storage enzyme can increase activity in the adipose cells.
3)	The energy cost of physical activity decreases as body weight decreases.

Prevention of obesity is important because only about 5% of people who diet lose weight and remain that weight. The evidence is strong that people can lose weight, but few can maintain that lower weight.

When dieters cut food intake, they often decrease salt intake. This slightly reduces fluid in the body. If the dieters reduce carbohydrate intake, this reduces glycogen stores in liver and muscles. Both factors contribute to an initial rapid weight loss.

1)	Reduce energy consumption.

2)	Alter problem behaviors that contribute to overweight and overeating.

3)	Increase physical activity.

A pound of fat tissue storage represents about 2700 to 3500 kcalories. Divided by 7 days, the dieter must reduce kcalories by about 400 to lose 1 pound per week, or 800 to lose 2 pounds per week. This is the limit of kcalorie reduction to still leave enough kcalories for obtaining an adequate diet.

Between 1500 to 1800 kcalories per day is the lowest recommendation. Below this kcalorie level women especially should consume some vitamin and mineral-fortified foods, such as fortified breakfast cereals, to obtain enough iron.

High-carbohydrate foods are the best foods because carbohydrates provide less than half as many kcalories as fat. In addition, high-carbohydrate foods are often bulky and therefore lead to a feeling of fullness.

Contrast direct and indirect calorimetry.

About how many kcalories are used each day for the thermic effect of food?

Briefly describe the three major categories of energy use by the body.

What physiological factors determine the rate of one's basal metabolism?

How much energy is used for this process?

Provide three suggestions for gaining weight for adults.

Does moderate obesity carry a social stigma it does not deserve, based on medical consequences?

Name five aspects of a good weight-loss diet.

What five types of behavior modification can help the weight loss process?

The thermic effect of food represents about 5% to 10% of kcalorie use. Given a 3000 kcalorie "Western" diet and using the 10% figure, this would account for 300 kcalories.

Both methods estimate energy use by the body. Direct calorimetry, measures the heat the body gives off. Indirect calorimetry measures oxygen consumption (or carbon dioxide output) and estimates the energy use associated with the use of that much oxygen.

One's rate of basal metabolism primarily depends on body surface area and lean body mass. A larger surface area and larger lean body mass yield a higher basal metabolism. A rough estimate is 1 kcalorie per minute, or 1440 kcalories per day.

<u>basal metabolism</u> -- the energy required to keep the resting body alive

<u>thermic effect of food</u> -- the increase in energy use associated with digestion, absorption, and metabolism of energy-yielding nutrients

<u>physical activity</u> -- any energy use for other than the two previous categories

---

You could argue "yes" in that the social stigma associated with being 20 to 30 pounds overweight is often much greater than the health consequences the extra weight brings.

---

1) The person could gradually increase consumption of kcalorie-dense foods, such as those higher in fat.

2) Higher-fat foods could be eaten at the end of the meal so they do not lead to early satiety.

3) Snacks made of dried fruits, bananas, nuts, and granola could be eaten regularly.

---

1)	chain breaking
2)	stimulus control
3)	cognitive restructuring
4)	contingency management
5)	self-monitoring

A good weight-loss diet will:
1) meet nutritional needs,
2) accommodate the dieter's habits and tastes, 3) include a range of readily obtainable foods, 4) promote changing habits that lead to overeating,
5) encourage an increase in physical activity.

Contrast hunger, appetite, and satiety.

How is body mass index calculated?

What is the cutoff value for obesity?

Provide a way to calculate a rough estimate for total energy needs.

What does the term desirable body weight mean?

Briefly describe three ways to determine the amount of body fat in a person.

What body shape is more closely associated with health risks from obesity?

What constitutes a "thrifty" metabolism?

In what ways might it be "thrifty"?

Provide an example for the effect of both nature and nurture on obesity.

Body mass index = weight in kilograms/height^2 in meters; values greater than 30 suggest obesity.

A desirable value is approximately 19-24.

---

 can be viewed as the physiological drive to find and eat food, whereas represents the more psychological drive to do so. should result from fulfilling hunger or appetite impulses because it represents a lack of desire to eat food.

A desirable body weight is estimated from the 1983 Metropolitan Life Insurance Table. This gives a body weight that is associated with maximum longevity.

Sedentary people need about 9 kcalories per pound of body weight. Light activity requires about 13 kcalories per pound. Heavy activity requires approximately 20 kcalories per pound.

Upper body (apple shape) obesity is more associated with health risks than the lower body (pear shape) obesity. Upper body distribution represents a waist to hip circumference ratio > 0.8 in women and > 0.95 in men.

Body fat can be estimated by:

1) measuring skinfold thickness in various sites in the body.

2) measuring the resistance of the body to electrical current using a bioelectrical impedance instrument.

3) underwater weighing is the most accurate but least used method.

For nature, identical twins raised apart tend to have similar weight gain patterns.

For nurture, men tend to become obese in middle age, whereas women tend to develop obesity during grade school years.

In the thrifty metabolism concept, some individuals naturally need less energy than others and therefore more easily gain weight and lose weight with more difficulty. A thrifty metabolism could be generated by less fidgeting or by an increased efficiency for synthesizing ATP.

When should a very low calorie diet (VLCD) be used to treat obesity?

What does it entail?

What is a "set point"?

How powerful is the set point for weight?

Define the term energy balance.

What role does the hypothalamus play in hunger regulation?

What is the basis behind behavior modification?

Simplify the terms stimulus control and contingency management.

What are two tip-offs that suggest a diet is a fad diet?

When is gastroplasty used to treat obesity?

What does it entail?

When using physical activity to help lose weight, what is the key factor on which to concentrate?

A "set-point" for weight refers to the day-to-day constancy of body weight. Factors tend to keep body weight constant, but statistics show that adults increase in body weight over 20 years . Thus the set point is not perfect.

A very low calorie diet (VLCD) could be considered if the person is 40% over desirable body weight and has failed more conventional diet approaches. The VLCD contains 400 to 800 kcalories and relatively little carbohydrate.

The hypothalamus has certain centers of cells that probably monitor the levels of energy-yielding nutrients, such as glucose, amino acids, and fatty acids in the bloodstream. A high level of energy-yielding nutrients leads to satiety; a low level leads to hunger.

Energy balance is the comparison of energy intake from foods versus energy output; it also considers changes in energy stores, as in fat stores. If a person's energy intake exceeds energy output, he/she will gain weight. If energy intake is less than output, weight will be lost.

Two possible tip-offs are:

1)	the promotion of quick weight loss. This is impossible if one is talking about fat loss

2)	there is no attempt to permanently change eating habits. The dieter follows the diet, loses the weight, and then returns to previous eating habits

The basic approach of behavior modification is to reshape one's environment so that weight maintenance, rather than weight gain, is the overwhelming thrust. Stimulus control refers to minimizing the factors in one's life that encourage overeating. Contingency management involves setting a plan to deal with diet lapses.

Duration is the key factor, rather than intensity. An activity should last long enough to burn 200 to 300 extra kcalories. That requires about 1 hour of brisk walking.

Gastroplasty is used to treat severe (morbid) obesity. (Recall that severe obesity is when a person weighs twice the desirable weight, or is 100 pounds overweight.) Gastroplasty calls for reducing the size of the stomach to approximately the size of a shot glass. This then limits meal size and reduces overeating.

CHAPTER 11

Define metabolism.

Outline anaerobic glycolysis and when it is used.

Give an example of an anabolic pathway.

List one ergogenic aid athletes use in an attempt to raise blood concentration of fatty acid. What is the overall purpose of this practice?

Give an example of a catabolic pathway.

Define the process of carbohydrate loading.

Briefly describe one advantage and one limitation of using the splitting of phosphocreatine to form ATP.

Why is it important to distinguish between high carbohydrate versus high fat meals for the athlete?

Anaerobic glycolysis is seen when the oxygen supply is limited or when exercise is intense. Glucose is broken down into a 3-carbon compound that accumulates in the muscles and is converted to lactic acid.

Metabolism is a term that encompasses all chemical processes in the body. In other words, it includes any sequence of chemical processes from beginning to end.

Consuming caffeinated beverages is one practice. This is done in an attempt to utilize more fat during prolonged exercise, thereby sparing muscle glycogen stores.

Anabolic -- build compounds using $O_2 + H_2O + CO_2$ in a specific way to form fatty acids, glucose or even complex cholesterol molecules.

Seven days prior to competition, consume 350 grams of carbohydrate per day. During the 72 hours prior to the event, 525-625 grams per day is recommended. A gradual decrease in exercise intensity is also recommended in the few days before competition.

Catabolic pathways lead to the breakdown of compounds into smaller units, such as when glucose and fatty acids are broken down into CO_2 and H_2O.

Fat won't make glycogen, but carbohydrate will.

Advantage: it can be activated instantly.

Limitation: there is not enough of it stored in the muscles to sustain a high rate of ATP resupply for more than a few minutes.

Outline a muscle bulking diet.

Define the term ergogenic aid and give some examples of those that have been supported by scientific evidence.

List three ways iron can be lost in the female athlete.

A physically active lifestyle can reduce many risks of chronic diseases. Give examples of those diseases.

Describe a pre-event meal.

Give three basic components every exercise program should consist of and the amount of time that should be spent on each.

Describe a post-event meal.

What is the recommended intake of a carbohydrate solution before and during exercise? Give amount and percentage for each.

Ergogenic (work-producing aids) are used to achieve better performance. Those that have documented scientific evidence include sufficient water, lots of carbohydrates, and a balanced diet.

During muscle building, athletes should consume 1 to 1.5 grams of protein per kilogram of body weight per day. This is slightly above the RDA of 0.8 grams/kilogram.

- cardiovascular heart disease

- diabetes

- obesity

- osteoporosis

1)	sweat

2)	foot-strike destruction of red blood cells.

3)	iron loss during menstruation

Warm-up:	5 to 10 minutes

Work-out:	20 or more minutes

Cool-down:	5 to 10 minutes

A pre-event meal should include a light meal eaten 2 to 4 hours before an endurance event to pay glycogen stores. The meal should consist of primarily complex carbohydrates, contain little fat or fiber, and include a moderate amount of protein.

Before:	1 to 2 cups of 10% to 20% CHO solution.

During exercise:	1/2 to 1 cup of a 5% to 8% CHO solution (like a sports drink) every 15 to 20 minutes.

A post-event meal should contain a large portion of carbohydrate. This should be consumed within 2 hours of the event, the sooner the better. Food such as candy, sugared soft drinks, and fruit juice can aid in reloading muscles with glycogen.

Is it possible to separate totally the diseases of anorexia nervosa and bulimia?

Define the term bulimia.

What is the hallmark of this disease?

What are the two major health problems associated with bulimia?

Define the term anorexia nervosa.

What is the hallmark of this disease?

Outline the treatment for bulimia.

Outline the basic treatment for anorexia nervosa.

List three potential health problems caused by anorexia nervosa.

What is the profile of the typical person with bulimia?

Bulimia is a disorder in which the person binges on large amounts of food and then tries to purge those kcalories by fasting, vomiting, exercise, or other means. The hallmark of the disease is the binge-purge cycle.

No, the diseases anorexia nervosa and bulimia considerably overlap. People with anorexia nervosa might go through stages of bingeing and purging, whereas those with bulimia might go through stages of semistarvation.

Anorexia nervosa is a psychological disorder in which the person loses significant amounts of weight and ends up essentially "skin and bones." The hallmark of the disease is a refusal to eat enough kcalories to support energy needs.

1) If the person purges by vomiting, teeth become demineralized and may require extraction.

2) The blood potassium level often decreases because vomit contains much potassium. This can cause problems in heart rhythm and even lead to sudden death.

Treatment of anorexia nervosa requires professional help, especially psychological therapy. In the initial stages, refeeding the person is important to regain physical energy and decrease the mental preoccupation with food.

Treatment for bulimia includes psychotherapy, primarily to help the person acquire a better sense of body image and self-image. The nutritional emphasis is on regular eating habits, not on stopping and bingeing and purging. Once regular eating habits are established, the bingeing and purging cycle should stop by itself.

The individual is usually a college-age woman and probably has been on many weight reduction diets since her teenage years. She is usually only slightly overweight.

Potential health problems include:
1) a decreased body temperature,
2) decreased heart rate, 3) anemia,
4) low white blood cell count,
5) constipation, 6) low blood potassium level, 7) a loss of menstruation, 8) bone loss, and
9) possibly heart failure.

Name three causes of death associated with anorexia nervosa.

What are three sources of false messages concerning the "ideal" body?

What are the three different methods of compulsive overeating?

What are two main factors that contribute to the onset of anorexia nervosa?

Repeated vomiting can have what three adverse affects on the body?

Nutritional counseling of a person with bulimia takes what approach, rather than focusing on stopping the bingeing and purging cycle?

What are the typical social characteristics of a person with anorexia nervosa?

What are aspects of the psychological profile?

Define the term baryophobia.

What causes this disease?

Sources include:

1) TV programs
2) billboard ads
3) magazines
4) movies
5) newspapers

---

1) suicide

2) heart ailments

3) infections

---

1) Adolescents' need for acceptance from parents and peers causes them to react intensely to how they think others perceive them.

2) Adolescent body changes are beyond the control of teens and they seek a way to keep control over their bodies.

---

1) continually eating over a defined period of time, called grazing

2) cycles of bingeing interspersed with normal eating

3) eating normally until an emotional setback occurs, and then large amounts of food is eaten

---

Setting up regular eating habits.

Affects of repeated vomiting include:

1) demineralization of teeth

2) lowered blood potassium levels that can disturb the heart's rhythm

3) swollen, infected salivary glands

4) stomach ulcers

5) tears in the esophagus

Baryophobia -- fear of fat -- is a relatively new disorder found in children and is characterized by poor growth. This poor growth usually results from parents underfeeding their children because they fear their children may develop early stages of heart disease or become obese.

The person generally comes from a higher socioeconomic class, may participate in physical activity such as ballet and gymnastics or work as a model. The person generally sees herself as fat, although she is thin, and often thinks her stomach protrudes.

CHAPTER 13

What is the difference between an embryo and a fetus?

What is the major difference between the diets for a pregnant and a breast-feeding woman?

How does the fetus receive nourishment?

What are two goals of a successful pregnancy that pertain to the infant?

When is the best time for a woman to focus on good nutritional habits to increase chances for having a healthy baby?

What are the two most important factors that influence infant birth weight?

What are three abnormalities seen in infants with fetal alcohol syndrome (FAS)?

Name two conditions that develop more frequently in low-birth-weight infants.

The breast-feeding diet is basically the same as that in pregnancy, with the exception of increased calcium, fluid, and kcalorie needs; an extra glass of milk suffices.

Embryo refers to human offspring from the time of conception to 8 weeks of gestation. After that point, the offspring is a fetus.

Two goals for a successful pregnancy regarding the infant are a gestational period longer than 37 weeks and a birth weight greater than 2500 grams (5-1/2 pounds).

The mother nourishes her offspring via the placenta.

Environmental factors such as smoking and nutritional factors, such as the mother's weight gain, have the most influence on birth weight outcome. Genetics has less of an effect.

Long before a woman becomes pregnant is the ideal time to focus on nutrition. Good nutritional practices are especially critical throughout a woman's childbearing years.

Low-birth-weight infants are at a great risk for infections, other illnesses, physical problems, and death.

Heavy or regular alcohol use during pregnancy can result in poor fetal and later infant growth, physical abnormalities, and mental retardation.

What is the most critical time period with respect to fetal development?

Why is fasting or "crash" dieting dangerous for fetal development?

How many additional kcalories are needed as a result of pregnancy?

What risk is increased by maternal smoking, alcohol consumption, imprudent medication use, and illicit drug use during pregnancy?

What is potentially harmful about the "eating for two" concept some pregnant women have?

What mineral need of pregnancy can only be met with a supplement?

What is the recommended weight gain during pregnancy?

Using the Food Guide Pyramid, outline a recommended diet during pregnancy.

A pregnant woman will develop ketosis if food intake is greatly restricted. Ketone bodies are thought to be poorly used by the fetal brain, and thus restrict brain development.

The first trimester is the most critical period for fetal development. Most organs show great development during this time.

These factors greatly increase the risk of having a premature or small-for-gestational-age infant.

Pregnancy demands an average 300 extra kcalories each day in the second and third trimesters.

Iron needs are so high that all women should take a prenatal iron supplement.

Although kcalorie and nutrient needs do increase, the mother does not have that many extra kcalories to use (about 300 per day in the second and third trimesters) for meeting these increased other nutrient needs.

An adequate diet during pregnancy should include the following servings from each food group:
4 - milk, yogurt, and cheese
2 to 3 - meat, poultry, fish, beans
2 to 4 - fruits
3 to 5 - vegetables
6 to 11 - breads, cereals, rice, pasta

The weight gain goal is 25 to 35 pounds for women of desirable body weight. The recommendation is adjusted for underweight and overweight women.

Name the vitamin that might need to be supplemented in the diet of a breast-fed infant.

What changes in food habits will ease the problem of constipation in pregnancy?

List two ways a pregnant woman can easily increase her folate intake.

What is the main factor that stimulates human milk production?

Name and describe the first fluid produced by the mother's breast.

Name the important reflex of the mother that is necessary for breast-feeding.

Why do breast-fed infants show typically fewer respiratory and intestinal infections than formula-fed infants?

How can a nursing mother know if her infant is receiving enough milk?

An increased intake of water, dietary fiber, and dried fruits, along with regular exercise, can help reduce constipation.

Although a form of vitamin D is present in human milk, supplementation is recommended <u>if adequate sunlight exposure cannot be guaranteed</u>.

Infant suckling stimulates the release of the hormone prolactin, which in turn stimulates milk production. The more the infant suckles, the greater is the production of milk.

Choosing folate-rich foods, such as oranges and other raw fruits and vegetables, as well as fortified breakfast cereals, helps meet folate needs. However, many physicians recommend a prenatal supplement to ensure adequate intake.

The "let down" reflex is necessary for the release of milk from storage so it can travel to the nipple.

Colostrum is the fluid produced for the first few days after birth. It is thick, yellowish, and contains immune factors.

A good standard is that the breast-fed infant should have at least six wet diapers a day and show normal growth.

The immune bodies present in colostrum and human milk compensate for the infant's immature immune system.

CHAPTER 14

How should new foods be added to an infant's diet to detect a possible allergy?

At what age do adolescent girls and boys experience a rapid growth spurt?

Name four common allergy-causing foods.

Compare the degree of hunger found in an infant to that found in a preschooler.

What should be the focus when assessing a teenager's snacking habits?

Name two ways parents can help their preschooler develop a healthful eating pattern.

Define the term food intolerance.

Why might a child benefit from being constantly introduced to new foods?

In most girls a growth spurt begins between the ages of 10 and 13 years, whereas in boys it begins between ages 12 and 15 years.

New foods should be introduced singly, not mixed, in 7-day intervals. This allows time to determine if an allergy develops and thus permits the offending food to be easily identified.

Preschoolers normally experience less hunger than they did as infants because of decreased growth rates.

Egg whites, chocolate, nuts, and cow's milk are the most common allergy-causing foods fed to infants.

Parents can set a good example by eating a variety of healthful foods. Encouraging the preschooler to take at least one bite of everything will help ensure variety in the diet.

Snacking is not inherently harmful; the focus should be on what makes up the snack. Wise food choices can make snacks a healthful part of a teenager's diet.

Providing new foods to a child can expand his or her food choices, help develop an experimental approach, and teach the child to enjoy a variety of foods.

A food intolerance is an adverse reaction to food that does not involve an immune process. Most people are less sensitive to their food intolerances than allergic people are to their offending foods.

What historical evidence suggests that nurture is very important for allowing maximal development?

At what age does a child first attempt self-feeding?

Why would inhibiting cell division, as can result from a poor diet, be so harmful?

Compare the protein needs of an infant with those of an adult on a per kilogram basis.

Which methods provide useful information on growth and development?

What unit of measurement is used for this method?

Compare the water need of an infant with that of an adult on a per kcalorie expended basis.

Describe how a food allergy is tested.

How can iron deficiency be prevented in childhood?

About 10 months of age is when an infant practices self-feeding of finger foods and drinking from a cup.

From suits of armor and Egyptian mummies we can tell that adults of the past were smaller than adults today, even though infants were the same size. The poor diets of people in the past did not supply enough nutrients for maximal growth.

Infants need 2.0 to 2.2 grams of protein per kilogram of body weight daily. This is more than twice the RDA for adults (0.8 grams per kilogram).

Improving the diet, once the time for cell division has stopped, will not restore any lack of growth experienced.

Infants need 1.5 milliliters of water per kcalorie expended or about 150 milliliters per kilogram of body weight. This is 1.5 times more than the needs of an adult (1 milliliter per kcalorie expended).

The height-for-age and weight-for-height growth charts give useful information in assessing growth and development. Numbers in these charts are expressed in percentiles, which represent the rank of the person among 100 age- and sex-matched peers.

Regular consumption of good iron sources is essential. A few ounces of lean meat and a serving of iron-fortified cereal are generally easy to incorporate into a child's diet.

The first step in detecting a food allergy is to keep a detailed record of symptoms, the time from ingestion to onset of symptoms, and suspected foods. Then all suspected foods are removed from the diet and reintroduced singly in small amounts.

What are two causes of failure to thrive?

How often should an infant be burped during breast- or bottle-feeding?

What four factors should be considered when deciding to introduce solid food to an infant's diet?

What is the greatest quantity of formula or milk infants should be fed daily?

At about what age should children be started on solid food?

At what age should bottle-feeding be discontinued?

What is one widespread reason for introducing solid foods earlier than the recommended time?

What is the best age and method to treat childhood obesity?

It is important to burp an infant every 10 minutes while breast-feeding or after 1 to 2 ounces while bottle-feeding.

Physical causes of failure to thrive include chronic diarrhea, infection, and heart problems. However, about half the cases show no disease process, and thus may result from poor child-rearing practices, such as inattention to the infant's needs.

Infants should not be fed more than 40 total ounces of formula or 32 total ounces of milk per day. After 6 to 8 months, solid foods in the diet should be increased instead.

One must consider 1) the infant's nutritional needs; 2) physiological readiness, such as kidney function and starch digestion; 3) physical readiness, such as sitting up and head control; and 4) susceptibility to allergies.

Bottle-feeding should be stopped by 18 months of age.

The American Academy of Pediatrics recommends that solid food not be given to infants until 4 to 6 months of age.

The best time to address obesity is in childhood because adolescent obesity most likely leads to adult obesity. The first step is to assess the child's activity level. Moderation in kcalorie intake is important; weight-loss diets are usually not necessary for young children.

Many people believe early introduction of solid food will help an infant sleep through the night. However, this ability is a developmental milestone and has little relation to what an infant eats before going to bed.

CHAPTER 15

Describe the autoimmune theory of cellular aging.

Why should many nutritional recommendations for health be individualized?

Name two significant drug-nutrient interactions that often exist in the elderly.

What have animal experiments with low-energy diets revealed about the link between aging and diet?

Describe our current understanding of the nutrient needs of the elderly.

Why is it important to make sure elderly people consume enough water?

Name three nutrients that deserve special emphasis in a diet plan for the elderly.

What is the main intestinal problem found in the elderly. How should it be treated with diet?

Since the response to different components is often idiosyncratic, dietary recommendations, such as for sodium and cholesterol, should be made on an individual basis to be most valid.

Autoimmune reactions occur when antibodies and white blood cells cannot distinguish between foreign compounds and your own body. Thus your immune system attacks your body tissue as well as foreign compounds. This can kill cells, and in turn lead to some effects of aging.

In experiments, animals that were raised on two-thirds of the energy they would normally consume lived 50% longer than those freely fed. This suggests that a slowing of the aging process may be linked to low-kcalorie diets.

Drug-related nutritional problems include an increased need for potassium when using some types of diuretics and changes in appetite when certain antibiotics are used.

Partial loss of the sense of thirst typically occurs among the elderly. This puts them at a greater risk for dehydration, which can lead to confusion.

Scientists have only recently started to study this area extensively. Most recommendations are made using extrapolations from adult needs.

Many elderly persons suffer from constipation. They should gradually increase their dietary fiber intake to 35 grams daily. Fluid intake should also increase to prevent intestinal blockage from the high-fiber intake.

The elderly need to emphasize adequate intakes of vitamin D (or sun exposure), vitamin B-6, vitamin B-12, vitamin C, thiamin, riboflavin, iron, calcium, and zinc.

What are the two principal causes of death in Western society today?

Name two examples of community nutrition programs for the elderly.

What two basic processes cause the aging of cells?

How is the immune system affected by aging and diet?

What two nutrients are needed for proper immune function?

Describe how both errors in DNA replication and damage by free radicals can cause cells to age.

How does lifestyle affect muscle mass throughout adult years?

What are four symptoms of Alzheimer's disease?

Nutritional problems in a person with alcoholism result from deficiencies of a variety of nutrients. Name four nutrients commonly deficient in persons with alcoholism.

Nutrition programs for the elderly include congregate meals where elderly people gather for lunch, home delivery of meals, food cooperatives, and programs of many social organizations.

Heart disease and cancer are linked with most deaths in contemporary Western society.

The immune system becomes less efficient with age; adequate protein and zinc intakes are needed to maximize its function. Consuming animal proteins is the best way to obtain these nutrients.

Aging of cells is probably a result of both automatic cellular changes and environmental influences.

Lifestyle partly determines the rate of muscle mass deterioration. An active lifestyle helps maintain muscle mass, whereas an inactive lifestyle causes a loss of muscle mass.

1) Enough errors are made in DNA replication to prevent the cell from producing the proteins necessary for functioning, and therefore the cell dies.

2) Free radicals can attack cell membranes and proteins, in turn leading to cell death.

Choose:
- vitamin A
- thiamin
- niacin
- vitamin B-6
- folate
- vitamin D
- vitamin C
- vitamin K

1) Personality change

2) Unreasonable fears

3) Outbursts

4) General forgetfulness

According to recent research, how do the RDAs compare to the best estimates of the needs of the elderly?

Define life expectancy.

What is the life expectancy for men and women in the United States?

Heart attack and stroke -- the major cause of death in all adults -- are caused primarily by atherosclerosis and high blood pressure. Define atherosclerosis and tell how it can be controlled.

What is osteoporosis and why is this commonly seen in the elderly?

How can it be prevented?

How can depression and mental state affect nutritional status?

List three practical suggestions for diet planning for single elderly people.

List four reasons good nutrition is such a benefit to the elderly.

What are the recommendations for alcohol intake established by the National Academy of Science's report on diet and health?

Life expectancy is the time an average person can expect to live. Life expectancy in America is 71 years for men and 78 for women.

For healthy elderly people, the RDA is probably too high for vitamin A, too low for protein (active elders), vitamin D, B-6, and B-12, and about right for the other nutrients.

Osteoporosis is the decline in bone density associated with aging. It most commonly occurs in women, especially after menopause. Meeting the RDA for calcium can help build and maintain density in some types of bones. However, estrogen therapy at menopause is the best way to prevent bone loss in the spine.

Atherosclerosis is the process of accumulating plaque in the arteries, reducing their elasticity, constricting blood flow, and consequently elevating blood pressure. Use diet (and possibly medications) to keep serum cholesterol below 200 milligrams per 100 milliliters and blood pressure within normal limits. Also, don't smoke.

1) If you have a freezer, cook large amounts, divide into portions, and freeze.

2) Ask the grocer to break open a family-sized package of wrapped meat or vegetables.

3) Buy only several pieces of fruit - perhaps a ripe one, a medium-ripe one, and a green one - so that they will ripen over a period of several days.

Depression can lead to a downward spiral in which poor appetite produces weakness that leads to even poorer appetite. The resulting poor nutritional state can produce further mental confusion, increased isolation, and loneliness.

The Committee recommends limiting consumption to the equivalent of less than 1 ounce of pure alcohol in a single day. This is equivalent to 2 cans of beer, 2 small glasses or wine, or 2 average cocktails.

1) It delays some disease progression
2) Improves management of existing diseases
3) Increases mental, physical and social well being
4) Decreases the need for and length of hospitalization

CHAPTER 16

Name the first three steps in the behavior change process.

Quick service foods are characteristically high in ___________?

Name the final two steps in the behavior change process.

Is it more effective to attempt to change behavior using small steps or to address the entire behavior change at once?

How can keeping a food diary help in the behavior change process?

Describe the term reinforcement.

Describe how a good behavior change plan evolves.

What four parts should be included in a behavior contract?

Fat

In behavior change, a person must:
1) become <u>aware</u> of the problem,
2) study the problem and develop a
<u>receptive frame of mind</u> for change,
and then 3) attempt a <u>trial change</u>.

Attempting a series of small and perhaps easier changes makes success with the big problem more attainable. The success with each step provides motivation.

A person must receive <u>positive reinforcement</u> for the new behavior in order to <u>adopt</u> it successfully into his or her lifestyle.

Reinforcement is a reaction by others in response to a person's behavior. Positive reinforcement entails encouragement; negative reinforcement entails criticism or penalty.

A food diary can be an effective tool for gathering baseline information about present behavior. Review of the diary may reveal patterns, associations, and areas that need improvement.

A behavioral contract should include:
1) a list of goal behaviors
2) objectives
3) ways to measure progress
4) regular awards for meeting the
   terms of the contract.

A good plan evolves from rational, deliberate decisions made after considering all options. All information at hand should be incorporated.

What are three primary and three secondary factors that drive our food choices?

List three ways to "psych yourself up" when encountering temptation to deviate from your behavior change plan.

Describe three steps for preventing behavior relapse.

What is the danger of setting the extinction of an unwanted behavior as a goal?

What is the benefit of having a trial period for a behavior change plan?

Describe the rationale behind avoiding problem situations in the early phases of behavior change.

What is contingency management?

Describe the term behavior chains.

1) Asserting yourself can help in many situations. Learn to say "no, thank you" to people and temptations.
2) In social situations practice choosing foods according to your plan, rather than other people's choices.
3) Practice stopping negative thoughts about yourself, focus on positive ones.

Sensory appeal such as flavor, appearance, and odor are most significant in directing food choices. Secondary factors include health value, expediency, energy value, and cost.

Striving for the extinction of a behavior may not be realistic. Focusing on reducing the frequency of the behavior may make a person less likely to become discouraged.

To prevent relapse:
1) identify high risk situations,
2) mentally rehearse a response to potential lapses, and
3) remind yourself of the original reasons for making the commitment to change.

Avoiding situations that are particularly tempting may be necessary at first until new habits are firmly established.

Contemplating a lifestyle change and the commitment involved may be initially overwhelming. Planning a 6- to 8-week trial period can make a goal seem more attainable and thus increase confidence.

Behavior chains are linked or related behaviors. It is important to control behavior chains that lead to the behavior one wants to change, such as visiting an all-you-can-eat restaurant and then overeating.

Contingency management involves planning in advance for failures so that when disruptive situations arise, one can react constructively.

How does the amount of an additive allowed in a food compare to the amount found safe in animal studies?

Name three naturally-occurring toxins in food.

What does the Delaney clause state?

How can variety and moderation in food selection protect against both naturally occurring and environmental food toxins?

Name two functions of antioxidants in foods.

What are three common antioxidants?

What responsibilities concerning food fall under the jurisdiction of the Food and Drug Administration (FDA)?

What are sulfites and why must they be specially regulated by FDA?

How does irradiation act to preserve food?

Some potentially harmful chemicals that occur naturally include aflatoxin, goitrogens, tannins, oxalic acid, solanine, and nitrates.

After scientists determine the highest dose of an additive that produces no ill effects in test animals, that amount is then divided by 100 to 1000 to establish the level allowed to be added to human food.

Variety and moderation in food selection help ensure that you are not consuming too much of any one food that may contain a contaminant. The frequency of exposure to any potentially toxin-laden food is thus decreased.

The Delaney clause prohibits the intentional use of cancer-causing compounds in food.

The Food and Drug Administration (FDA) ensures the safety and wholesomeness of all foods sold through interstate commerce, except for meat and poultry, which are under USDA jurisdiction. FDA sets standards and then enforces the regulations.

Antioxidants help delay discoloration of foods and help prevent fats from becoming rancid. BHA, BHT, and vitamins E and C are widely used antioxidants.

Food irradiation creates free radicals in food, which can destroy cell membranes and attack DNA and proteins. By doing so, irradiation can prevent the growth of microorganisms, parasites, and insects.

Sulfites and sulfur-containing compounds that prevent food discoloration. However, since some people are sensitive to sulfites and react with wheezing, hives, diarrhea, and other symptoms, FDA has prohibited their use on raw fruits and vegetables, except potatoes.

Describe how <u>Salmonella</u> bacteria usually enter foods.

Can refrigeration stop the growth of all bacteria?

In what temperature range should cooked foods be stored?

Name three methods of food preservation that have been used for centuries.

What treatment is recommended for diarrhea associated with food-borne illness?

What are the two basic ways in which food spoils?

Name three types of preservatives.

Describe the action of emulsifiers in foods.

No, some bacteria can grow even at refrigeration temperatures.

Salmonella bacteria are found in human and animal feces and enter the food chain via infected water, contaminated cutting boards, cracked eggs, and pieces of feces in food.

Past methods of food preservation include use of smoke, salt, sugar, fermentation, and drying.

Store cooked foods below 40° F (4° C) or above 140° F (60° C). This helps avoid holding foods in the moderate temperature range in which microbes flourish.

Food spoilage can occur from:

1)	bacterial, viral, or fungal contamination, or

2)	exposure to oxygen.

The person with diarrhea should drink plenty of fluids. To prevent further contamination, hands should be washed frequently and food handling should be temporarily avoided or at least minimized.

Emulsifiers suspend fat in water, preventing their separation. This often improves uniformity, texture, and body of a food.

Preservatives may be in the form of:

1)	antioxidants
2)	antimicrobials--inhibitors of microbial growth
3)	sequestrants -- these bind free metal ions

In what environment does <u>Clostridium botulinum</u> thrive?

Contrast intentional and incidental food additives.

Why are signs of spoilage on commercially canned foods, such as rust on seams, holes, and swollen sides, so dangerous?

What precautions should be taken if such spoilage is seen?

What is the GRAS list?

Why was it established?

Define the term pasteurization.

Which causes the greatest health risk from the food we eat: microbes or additives?

What two mechanisms do bacteria use to cause food-borne illness?

Describe how <u>Staphylococcus aureus</u> usually enters foods.

Intentional additives are directly and purposefully put into food. Incidental additives are those that may reasonably be expected to become components of food during processing or packaging. Both are regulated by FDA.

Clostridium botulinum are anaerobic bacteria and thus can only grow in absence of air. Improperly home canned food and foods with an anaerobic center, such as potato salad, can become contaminated.

The generally recognized as safe (GRAS) list was established in 1958 by the U.S. Congress. All food additives in use in the U.S. that were considered safe were put on the list so manufacturers would not needlessly have to prove their safety.

Signs of spoilage in commercially canned foods may indicate contamination by the anaerobic bacteria Clostridium botulinum. Do not taste the food. If Clostridium botulinum is present, the toxins could cause a fatal result.

Contamination by bacteria, and to a lesser extent by molds, fungi, and viruses, poses the greatest health risk from food.

Pasteurization is a partial sterilization process that uses high temperatures for a short time to destroy microorganisms.

Staphylococcus aureus bacteria live in nasal passages and the skin. When people sneeze or cough over food, or people with open sores handle food, the bacteria can enter the food.

Bacteria can either:

1)	directly invade the intestine in turn introducing toxins that are part of the cells themselves.

2)	produce toxins to cause food-borne illness.

CHAPTER 18

Describe three critical periods in human development.

Define the term malnutrition.

Define the term undernutrition.

This is mainly linked to what social factor?

Define the term protein-energy malnutrition.

Name five symptoms of chronic undernutrition.

What does the World Health Organization (WHO) mean by the term "silent undernutrition"?

List four factors that currently contribute to undernutrition in the Third World.

Describe the School Breakfast and Lunch programs.

Malnutrition is a condition of impaired development or function caused by a long-term deficiency, excess, or imbalance of kcalories, nutrients, or both.

Critical periods are times when the human organism is particularly susceptible to the effects of undernutrition because of rapid growth. These include pregnancy, infancy, and childhood.

Protein-energy malnutrition is a form of undernutrition caused by an extremely deficient intake of kcalories, protein, or both.

Undernutrition is the malnutrition that results from an inadequate intake, absorption, or utilization of the nutrients or kcalories needed for optimal growth, development, and body function.

Poverty is its major cause.

The term "silent undernutrition" is reflected in the young child whose weight is several pounds below the low end of the normal range on a growth chart. The untrained eye may miss this condition or simply see him or her as a skinny child.

---

1. tiredness

2. muscle soreness

3. irritability

4. edema

5. hunger pains

Both the School Lunch and Breakfast Programs enable low-income schoolchildren to receive meals at reduced cost or no cost if certain income guidelines are met.

---

1. inadequate food supplies
2. depletion of natural resources
3. poor infrastructure for food production and health maintenance
4. war or civil unrest
5. external debt
6. cultural attitudes towards certain foods

Describe the special supplemental feeding program for Women, Infants, and Children (WIC).

What did Thomas Malthus predict about the eventual course of the food/population ratio?

Outline a key step to ending hunger worldwide.

Define the term "green revolution".

Name four benefits of using breast milk for infant feeding in Third World countries.

Name three reasons for poor sanitation conditions in Third World countries.

Define the term biotechnology.

Name three aims of low input sustainable agriculture.

Malthus predicted the population would always increase in a geometric ratio -- 2, 4, 8, 16, 32, etc. -- while the food supply would increase only arithmetically -- 2, 4, 6, 8, 10, etc. This means that the population will eventually outgrow the food supply.

The WIC program provides food vouchers and nutrition education to low-income pregnant and lactating women and their young children.

The term "green revolution" describes a phenomenon starting in the 1960s where a dramatic rise in crop yields in some countries, such as the Philippines, India, and Mexico, was made possible because of increased use of fertilizers and development of superior crops through careful plant breeding.

Providing employment opportunities for all who desire to work is a key step to ending hunger worldwide.

---

1.   human feces

2.   rotting garbage

3.   insect and rodent infestations

Breast milk is hygienic, is readily available, nutritionally sound and provides immune factors.

---

1.   reduction in pesticide use

2.   reduction in fertilizer use

3.   less water and soil erosion

Biotechnology, which includes genetic engineering, uses a wide range of cells and subcell technology for synthesizing and then placing genetic material in organisms.